At one time allergies were thought of as [illegible] unusual phenomena, however as more radical forms of medicine come to light, this is no longer the case. Most of us have at least one or two allergies: the result of our environment caused by either food or chemicals. If we continue with our poor diets and the pollution of our surroundings, it is probable that we will all be affected by allergies to some degree.

Such is the premise of this book, which explains allergies and their possible solutions in terms of *clinical ecology*, rather than conventional medicine's traditional emphasis on drugs and surgery.

Dr Mumby explains in detail the most recent theories about allergy causes and effects; reviews all available current diagnoses and testing methods; and offers sound advice on self-help, and where to go for further information.

This is a complete guide, suitable for lay readers and professionals alike. It uses clear and straightforward language and, by enabling us to understand the principles of allergies, points to how both sufferers and non-sufferers alike can maintain better health in an increasingly complex and toxic world.

Dr Mumby is a doctor of medicine who runs a busy clinic in Manchester devoted entirely to allergy treatment.

Also by Keith Mumby and published by
Unwin Paperbacks

The Food Allergy Plan

Allergies ...what everyone should know.

Keith Mumby MB, ChB

London
UNWIN PAPERBACKS
Boston Sydney

First published by Unwin Paperbacks 1986

UNWIN® PAPERBACKS
40 Museum Street, London WC1A 1LU, UK

Unwin Paperbacks
Park Lane, Hemel Hempstead, Herts HP2 4TE, UK

Allen & Unwin Australia Pty Ltd
8 Napier Street, North Sydney, NSW 2060, Australia

Unwin Paperbacks with the Port Nicholson Press
PO Box 11-838 Wellington, New Zealand

British Library Cataloguing in Publication Data

Mumby, Keith
Allergies: what everyone should know.
1. Allergy
I. Title
616.97 RC584

ISBN 0-04-641048-1

Typeset in 10 on 11 point Sabon by
Mathematical Composition Setters Ltd, Salisbury
Printed and bound in Great Britain by
Cox & Wyman Ltd, Reading

The doctor of the future will give no medicine but will interest his patient in the care of the human frame, in diet, and in the cause and prevention of disease.

Thomas Edison, inventor, genius.

Contents

Introduction

This book is based on the belief that allergies are very common. In fact, probably most people have one or two, though not necessarily to the extent that could be called illness. The trouble is the problem is getting worse and it is going to get *much* worse unless we stop polluting our environment haphazardly and irresponsibly with drugs, agricultural chemicals, industrial effluvia and toxic waste. Probably it is no exaggeration to state that sooner or later we shall all be ill. The warning signs are all there for those who know what to look for. Deterioration in body defenses, especially immunity, due to cumulative poisoning is only one aspect of the environmental pollution problem but it is an important one and something that *everyone* should be concerned about: hence the title.

The subject of allergies (or, as you will read, the larger umbrella of clinical ecology) is very much in the public eye. Newspapers and television have on numerous occasions made a feature of this or that startling case of recovery brought about by the simple expedient of eliminating allergenic foods from the diet or by other modifications of environment and lifestyle. These cases are indeed the stuff of human drama, the sort of stories that make good media, especially if, as is so often the case, the reports are able to poke fun at the apparent incompetence of conventional medicine which failed to help. Doubtless this fad will pass, as do so many other media fashions. But when all the fuss has died down, what we are left with is the fact that there has been a revolution in medicine which promises to be as far-reaching as the development of antisepsis, anaesthesia and antibiotics.

Admittedly 'underdeveloped' countries have their own frightful health problems but certainly in our Western society, where the principal infectious diseases are under control, illnesses caused by dietary and environmental factors have now moved very much to the fore. Such illnesses include allergies but actually there is a far wider significance, covering such powerful hazards as cancer and heart disease, which seem to have very important dietary and environmental causes (though these causes are *not* allergies).

The startling fact is that, despite all the advances in knowledge, ignorance and mis-information are abundant. Even doctors themselves seem bewildered and uncertain as to what point of view to take. Some seem to want to ignore the subject or underplay it; some want to attack it though, interestingly, I haven't met a doctor hostile to the methods given in this book who has actually taken the trouble to apply them! Few it seems have troubled to make the effort to learn about the new discoveries and use them to help their sick patients.

Viewed in terms of the amount of illness, which is growing, and the number of people on chronic drug treatment, which amounts to a lack of a cure, modern medicine is a failure. Yet the established order always has the most influence and that makes educating the public and profession much more difficult. Undeterred, I embarked on this second book concerning allergies, which is an attempt to explain the causes, the hazards and most importantly the treatments of allergy as succinctly as possible. It is anticipated that my principal readership will come from the lay population, though hopefully the book will also find its way on to the bookshelf in one or two surgeries. Accordingly, I have kept the descriptions and language as simple and non-technical as possible.

Some of the material has been duplicated from my earlier book *The Food Allergy Plan* (Unwin Paperbacks, London, 1985). This is in order that the present volume can stand complete on its own. Thus for example the table of symptoms in chapter 3 is reprinted for those who wish to assess themselves in regard to environmental illness. Also several addresses in the appendix have been repeated as they are extremely pertinent. Chapter 4 is almost a synopsis of my first book, but no book on allergies would be complete or comprehensible without details of detecting food allergy by means of dietary manipulation. I hope those who read both books will bear with me in this.

Obviously it has not been possible to give a comprehensive overview in a volume this size but I have tried to cover the ground as lucidly and informatively as possible, without ducking too many issues. At the same time I have tried to be reasonably objective but, when all is said and done, writing is a pleasure instead of a chore only if one is allowed to express one's own opinion now and again! The important thing is for the reader to recognise opinions for what they are and not to be unduly swayed by them. The book is not intended to be a definitive work but simply a guide, bearing in mind that our knowledge of the subject is changing and advancing so rapidly, that it would not be appropriate to be too dogmatic.

I hope, however, you enjoy the book and find it useful. If you are ill and possibly in despair, it is my earnest wish that you find something in these pages that will lead you to a successful recovery.

Happy reading.

1

Who Gets Allergies?

Until recently it was held that allergic reactions were rare, especially allergic reactions to food. Most people have heard of dust and feathers causing diseases such as asthma attacks, and of course hay-fever, the bane of English summers, affects so many people that allergy to pollen could never be considered rare. Nonetheless, despite these acknowledged instances, and the realisation that some unfortunate people suffer with rashes after eating strawberries or shellfish, nobody – not even the majority of doctors – considered allergy a major factor in ill-health.

Lately this has been changing, due to the efforts of a small but dedicated group of doctors who call themselves clinical ecologists. Notwithstanding the indifference and even scorn of their medical colleagues they have blazed a new trail in therapeutics, studying in great detail the way in which our environment is making many of us ill. They have been proclaiming loudly for some time that allergies, far from being rare, are a major cause of illness in our time. This includes particularly diseases caused by reactions to food. *Allergies probably now account for over 50 per cent of all health problems in Western society. Foods are a major cause, but environmental pollution is also a deadly cause of disease for many of us.* Some workers put the percentage much higher.

As conditions caused by bacteria, viruses and parasites come under control, we are left with the realisation that many illnesses are caused by factors in the environment, which have no effect on the majority of us (at least not so far as we know) but make some people very sick indeed. Previously the role of these disease agents was little known and poorly understood. Certainly, the extent of the problem was not recognised until recently. Even now, we do not understand the real mechanisms involved, but at least we can, and should, remain aware of the existence of the problem and in the meantime try to help sufferers by identifying and removing these hostile factors. Unfortunately many doctors have not even got that far in their thinking.

Many chemicals are present in our environment, some are plentiful, despite known toxicity. It is hardly surprising that these should be the cause of symptoms and disease; the evidence is abundant that this is so, despite official cant and blithe reassurances to the contrary.

The problem is not confined to poisonous chemicals. Diet is to blame far more often. Some foods, as you will read, can in certain situations act as poisons. This even includes whole fresh food, such as raw milk, fruit, wholemeal bread and much else. Then there are food additives – artificial chemicals, many of which, if not the majority, are unquestionably inimical to some of us, and which for commercial advantage are introduced into what we eat. Do not be reassured by the standard government line: so-called safety limits are based on little or no knowledge, inadequate and out-dated tests, bias, vested interest, and outright incompetence. The IBT scandal (in which an official US government drug and chemical safety testing agency was found to be falsifying results) and its shock waves have rocked what little faith there was in government-authorised testing and the reliance on standard tests as a criterion of safety. Reflect for a moment that there are over 1,100 chemicals listed as 'safe' in the UK, yet in France there are less than a dozen. Does this not suggest the possibility that we are being told that well over a thousand chemicals are safe to add to our food when they are not? At least the French authorities think they are not. So do doctors like myself.

Cancer is believed to be caused, or strongly influenced, by chemicals in our diet, air and water supplies. Considering this disease is so much on the increase and most available treatment almost as frightful as the affliction itself, that makes deliberate contamination of our diet seem incautious in the extreme. Yet we go on permitting it. It is not the purpose of this book to argue that cancer is produced by allergic reactions, although at this stage nobody can claim evidence to the contrary either. But allergic reactions can be a form of illness in themselves, and they can be caused by food additives.

Ecology is a fashionable word. It was first coined by Haeckel in 1866, and means the study of an organism's interrelationship with its environment. Hence 'clinical ecology', the study of the ways in which environment makes us ill. Practitioners feel somewhat uncomfortable about this label, believing it may be associated in people's minds with radical ecological and 'peace' movements of the political type. Nevertheless, to date no better alternative has suggested itself. It is a new discipline in medicine and not an 'alternative'. Despite the fact that the majority of members of the medical profession have not yet awakened to its vital and urgent message, with its implications for us all, it remains properly the domain of the qualified medical practitioner, who can use its valuable data in conjunction with existing medical knowledge.

If you need help personally, go to your own doctor armed with this book and insist that he act. In the unlikely event that he or she refuses to help, seek out the aid of a practising clinical ecologist by contacting an action group such as Action Against Allergy.

A recent and disconcerting trend (partly made possible, perhaps, due to frustration at the slowness of the medical profession in accepting these new ideas) is exemplified by the appearance of a number of non-qualified people, some with doctorate of philosophy degrees (PhDs), who are setting themselves up and calling themselves 'doctor' and purporting to treat allergies along the lines given in this book. Sometimes they have no qualifications at all, other than an amateurish enthusiasm. Such people are legally entitled to do this but they are *not* entitled to allow patients mistakenly to think that they are *medical* doctors, which is misrepresentation. It may be old-fashioned to talk of quackery, but if you want your Rolls-Royce car serviced you would naturally go to a Rolls-Royce-trained engineer, not a general mechanic or, even worse, an odd-job man.

This is not to say that a great deal of useful work cannot be done by interested allied workers, such as dieticians, or that it isn't an area in which we cannot all be involved. The dissemination of knowledge is vital and is everyone's concern. It would be less embarrassing for me to make these points if my fellow doctors were not so resistant to this new methodology.

Fortunately there are signs that it is being accepted slowly by my colleagues, as you will read. It is worth remembering that it took over thirty years for the idea that bacteria can cause disease to be accepted. There is a peculiar stubborn streak among doctors that renders them insensitive to new ideas, even when these new ideas would mean better treatment for patients.

HOW COMMON ARE ALLERGIES?

As stated previously, this book is predicated on the knowledge that allergies are *very* common. This idea is not widely accepted, but that is due simply to the fact that previously no one knew what to look for. The clues are obvious and widespread, once understood. By the time you have finished this book, you will be aware of ample evidence of at least minor allergic reactions amongst your family and friends. Perhaps you are manifesting a few yourself.

The dividing line between an important and an unimportant allergy is whether or not it constitutes an illness. Most complaints are trivial and the sufferer would not ordinarily consult a doctor because of them. Though there is always the disconcerting possibility that these may get worse and develop into serious disease. Not everyone suffering from an allergy becomes ill in the strict sense of the word. As Dr E. C. Hamlyn of Ivybridge, Devon, puts it, 'There are many people with a few allergies and a few people with a lot of allergies.' It is this latter group who become medical cases. But the fact remains there are very many of us who could lead happier and healthier lives by understanding and correcting environmentally induced reactions.

Dr Arthur Coca, an American allergist, estimated that 90 per cent of the population has at least one food allergy.[1] Locke, in a statistical study, placed it nearer to ninety-five per cent. I repeat, an allergy does not necessarily imply illness. Suffering indigestion or flatulence as a result of eating onion or bananas does not constitute a disease. But it is an allergy of sorts.

Indirect evidence concerning the frequency of allergies was collected in 1984 by Dr Vicky Rippere of the London Institute of Psychiatry. Normal individuals, by which is meant those who had not seen their doctor for any treatment in the previous twelve months, were asked to fill out a questionnaire. This included a list of symptoms similar to the one in Chapter 3, which are suggestive of allergic disorder. Any one symptom may have a number of causes but taken together, the more symptoms are present, the more certain it is that some degree of allergic sensitivity exists.

Results showed that forty-six people suffered an astonishing total of 422 symptoms between them. Sixty-seven per cent had five or more such symptoms, 41 per cent had ten or more. Remember these are 'healthy' people. One had thirty-two separate symptoms and yet did not consider this abnormal!

The table below summarises the most frequently complained of symptoms:

TABLE 1.1 FREQUENCY OF ALLERGIES

Symptom	*Sufferers: as percentage of group*
over- or under-weight	52
headache	50
irritability	47
feeling low/depressed	32
lack of energy	30
red or itchy eyes	28
insomnia	26
menstrual difficulties	26
abdominal bloating	26
flatulence	26
runny/blocked nose	24
persistent fatigue	17
aching joints	17
occasional swellings of face, hands and abdomen	17

Remember this is an empirically derived list of symptoms. They are encountered over and over again in allergic patients. What is much more important is that symptoms like these will tend to *disappear* when allergens are located and removed from the person's diet or environment. Hence the belief that they are representative of induced reactions to badly tolerated foods and chemicals. Chapter 3 has more details.

Naturally, open studies of this kind are not considered scientifically valid. Certainly, they are not conclusive in any sense of the word. But it can hardly be denied that the results point to the existence of a very significant problem.

WHO SUFFERS WITH ALLERGIES?

We might also ask ourselves what type of individual or group is most likely to have a predisposition towards allergic reactions, to have what is known as an allergic diathesis. No significant demographic study exists which takes in all the parameters of ecologically-based illness. It is not possible, for example, to say that one social class is more significantly affected than others. The absence of such research is partly due to lack of resources, and partly to lack of interest by any research group, but principally it is due to lack of any definite criteria by which to carry out the investigation. Thus we are left with the tentative approaches of the few individuals quoted above.

We know from related studies that all nutritionally-based illnesses are at their worst in social class 5 (the working class). There is an unfortunate economic pressure today to eat badly, especially high allergy-risk foods (you will learn later which these are). Bad diet unquestionably leads to illness; it was, for example, one of the major factors in the mortality rate of tuberculosis sufferers. Our modern, comparatively well-nourished, population is today less prone to this disease than were our ancestors, for whom the disease constituted a very real threat. Allergy is simply one other aspect of this nutritional blight. It costs money to eat properly, which is one of the great social evils of our age.

Speaking purely anecdotally, few doctors who understand the problems of environmentally-caused disease would deny that city-dwellers are significantly more at risk. The reason for this is atmospheric pollution. Allergic illnesses are cumulative. The body can cope amazingly well with the many insults it has to endure but there is a limit to what it can deal with. If this limit is exceeded, symptoms will inevitably result. Dr Richard Mackarness likens this effect to a barrel: food allergies, stress, atmospheric pollution, drugs and other affronts to the organism are represented by water flowing into this barrel – if the input is too much, it will overflow, which represents the symptoms.[2] Someone with a tendency to be made ill because of a sensitivity to foods is going to have a much worse time if he or she lives in an urbanised industrial area rather than by the sea, where the air is clean. Countless clinical observations support this fact, even your own experience on holiday may bear it out, but once again no proper scientific studies have been done. Useful available money which could be spent on this sort of research is disappearing into the coffers of drug companies, poured in by a health system which encourages doctors to take the easy way out and to continue writing prescriptions, instead of thinking things through.

MY OWN CLINIC

To give an idea of the broad diversity of cases, ages and types who suffer from allergies, I have listed fifty-four consecutive successful cases from the files of my own clinic. All unsuccessful cases have been left out. This is not through vanity, but simply to make the point that the cases quoted definitely did have the sort of problem we are discussing in this book – otherwise, presumably, they would not have recovered. Successful, by the way, does not necessarily mean a complete cure but in all cases the condition responded and the patient was significantly helped. I chose consecutive cases to give an element of 'randomness' to the series. Obviously one cannot infer that this is a scientific study, it is merely intended to sketch a picture.

As you can see there is a wide range of occupational and social types, in diseases that were suffered from and in agents that had been causing the trouble.

The very high incidence of women patients might be surprising to some. In fact, women outnumber the men by four to one. It must be assumed therefore that either women are more prone to this type of illness, or that they are more complaining by nature. The latter may be partly true, in a non-pejorative way, in that women seem to take their health more seriously and are less inclined to minimise or ignore symptoms. As one patient put it (a woman, of course) men are perhaps more afraid of self-knowledge and finding out the truth about their illnesses.

TABLE 1.2

Patient No.	*Sex*	*Age*	*Occupation*	*Presenting complaint*	*Discovered allergens**
1	female	13	student	sinusitis	**house dust**, **milk**, **egg**, **wheat**, **potato**
2	female	42	housewife	respiratory complaints	egg, coffee, tomato, chocolate
3	female	39	housewife	feeling faint; tinnitus	**potato**, **wheat**, **corn**, **milk**, **egg**, **tea**, cane sugar, **tomato**, **plaice**, **pork**
4	female	68	retired	sore throat; double vision and distortion	**wheat**, **corn**, **milk**, pineapple, rye, cheese, lamb
5	male	13	student	eczema; hyperactivity	**potato**, **pork**, **orange**, **cane sugar**, milk, egg, tea
6	female	41	social worker	stiff knees; inflamed eyes; psychological effects; no energy	**cheese**, **chocolate**, **oats**, rye, **carrot**, **yeast**, **tea**, **house gas**, **orange**, **formaldehyde**, **rice**, **tomato**, **apple**, wheat, **milk**, potato
7	female	31	infant teacher	depression; fatigue	**beef**, **rice**, **milk**, **wheat**, **egg**, orange
8	female	16	student	swelling and stiffness in joints	car exhaust, potato, chocolate, tomato

TABLE 1.2 (*Cont.*)

Patient No.	*Sex*	*Age*	*Occupation*	*Presenting complaint*	*Discovered allergens* *
9	female	35	hairdresser	migraine	**egg, milk, cheese, wheat**
10	male	4 yrs 10 mths		type of asthma	**wheat, milk, rice, house dust, house-dust mite, egg, yeast**
11	male	40	chartered surveyor	lack of concentration; depression; eczema; bowel trouble	**milk, egg, yeast, potato, wheat, coffee, car exhaust**
12	male	47	industrial chemist	fatigue; aching muscles and joints	**egg, cane sugar, beet sugar, peas, cabbage, coffee,** tobacco, cheese
13	female	54	receptionist	painful joints; tired and lethargic	milk, yeast, egg, cheese
14	female	10		migraine; headache; cystitis symptoms; eczema	**yeast, chicken, phenol, wheat, cheese, corn, house dust, house-dust mite**
15	female	55	conveyances legal executive	rheumatism	**wheat, corn, milk, tea, beef,** potato
16	female	40	assembler, packer	sinus trouble; asthma; bronchitis; arthritis, eczema	**house dust, house-dust mite, milk, tobacco, cheese, wheat, cane sugar, mould**

17	female	43	singer and violin teacher	catarrh and sore throats	**tea**, **house gas**, egg, cane sugar, house dust, car exhaust, lamb, pork
18	male	36	sales engineer	migraine	**corn**, **formaldehyde**, **cane sugar**, **milk**, banana, tea
19	female	23	media assistant	diarrhoea	**milk**, egg, chicken, beef, chocolate
20	female	16	student	itching and rashes; tiredness and flu-like symptoms	**corn**, **house dust**, **house-dust mite**, **horsehair**, pork, egg, milk, wheat, yeast
21	female	51	secretary	general malaise	**phenol**, **house gas**, **house-dust mites**, wheat, milk, yeast, tea, coffee, lamb, formaldehyde
22	female	48	housewife	painful joints	**potato**, **beef**, egg, yeast
23	female	32	education welfare officer	red blister rash	**milk**, egg, tea, **phenol**
24	female	39	clerk	chest trouble	**house dust**, **house-dust mite**, **wheat**, **milk**, **coffee**, **tomato**, **cheese**
25	male	45	bank official	arthritis of left hip	**wheat**, milk, egg, tea
26	male	13		bouts of vomiting and intermittent headaches	**wheat**, **milk**, **egg**, **potato**, **yeast**, **chicken**, **pollen** (some), **pork**

TABLE 1.2 (*Cont.*)

Patient No.	*Sex*	*Age*	*Occupation*	*Presenting complaint*	*Discovered allergens**
27	female	57	housewife	high blood pressure	**milk, egg, cane sugar, house gas, cheese, petrol exhaust**
28	male	4		hay fever symptoms	mould, house-dust mites, house dust, **wheat, potato, tomato**
29	female	33	housewife	headaches; depression	**milk, cane sugar, beet sugar,** beef, **apple**
30	male	2		sleeping problems; listlessness; irritability	**wheat, cane sugar, beet sugar**
31	male	5		headaches; bladder problems	**wheat, potato, tomato,** milk
32	male	25	photo litho retoucher	hay fever; dust allergy	cheese, potato, egg, milk, exhaust fumes
33	male	14		feeling off colour; aches and pains	**egg, pears, corn,** milk, pork, barley, lentils, nuts
34	female	30	housewife	fear of going out – meeting people; nervous symptoms	**yeast, tea, cheese, house gas, mould,** tomato, milk

35	female	48	housewife	eyes swelling	**formaldehyde**, **pork**, carrot, wheat
36	male	26	software engineer (computers)	asthma and dermagraphism	**egg**, **tea**, **yeast**, **potato**, tobacco
37	male	4 yrs 10 mths		frequent ear infections; nose trouble; face and ear pain, rashes	**cane sugar**, **car fumes**, **potato**, egg, beet sugar
38	male	3yrs 6 mths		cyclic periods of tiredness	wheat, corn, egg
39	female	37	housewife	sinus trouble; throat trouble; nausea and dizziness	**phenol**, **egg**, **cane sugar**, **cheese**, tea, wheat, milk, corn
40	male	43	dental surgeon	urticaria	mould, wheat, egg, grass, pine
41	male	34	engineer	ulcerative colitis; high blood pressure	**wheat**, **potato**, pineapple
42	female	36	teacher	sinusitis; rashes; depression; insomnia; headaches; unable to lose weight	**wheat**, **corn**, **milk**, egg, tea, potato, house dust, house-dust mite, orange

TABLE 1.2 (*Cont.*)

Patient No.	*Sex*	*Age*	*Occupation*	*Presenting complaint*	*Discovered allergens**
43	female	32	teacher	headaches; skin complaints; hay fever	**wheat, corn, egg, yeast, tobacco, tomato, cigarette smoke, potato, cheese**
44	female	42	market trader	always feeling ill; tired; irritable	**phenol, corn, egg, onion,** milk, tomato, pork
45	female	61	housewife	beginnings of osteo-arthritis	**pineapple, yeast, house gas, cane sugar, wheat,** lemon, egg
46	female	57	housewife	eczema	yeast, mould, lamb, chicken, egg, pineapple
47	female	25	housewife	eczema	milk, egg, tea, peas, apple, house dust, house-dust mite
48	female	25	teacher (junior)	depression; apathy; weakness	**wheat, potato, egg, tea,** formaldehyde, orange, grape, cheese
49	female	41	accountant	psoriasis	wheat, milk, egg, beef, lamb, cheese
50	female	17	bank clerk	skin disorders	**wheat, corn, coffee**
51	male	7		irritability; lack of concentration; bad behaviour; hay fever	**grass, mould,** coffee

52	male	46	insurance superintendent	fatigue and depression	**wheat, corn, milk, rye, pork, tomato, cane sugar, cheese, beef**
53	female	33	unemployed	feeling unsociable at times; weeping; rash on face; itchy eyes	potato, tea, tomato, coffee, onion
54	male	25	building contractor	fatigue; lack of concentration; unable to do physical work	**house gas, bath water, coffee,** onion, chocolate, yeast, **diesel fumes**
55	female	55	music teacher; composer	arthritis	**corn, milk, mould,** wheat, potato, lamb, house dust, house-dust mite, coffee

* Main allergies are set in bold type.

But it seems without question that women are truly more sensitive to food and chemical intolerances than men are. I have no direct proof but I believe this is due to the great stress laid on women's bodies by the constantly changing hormone levels. Indirectly, this is supported by the fact that at the principal crisis times of a woman's life, puberty, the menopause and to a lesser extent monthly periods, allergy-related illnesses often become much more pronounced. Presumably the body can't cope with food and chemical intolerances *and* put up with dramatic changes in internal physiology at the same time.

Pre-menstrual tension isn't new but the disconcerting extent of the problem is very much a phenomenon of our age, with its fast food and pollution. The fact is that few women can claim no loss of optimum mental and physical well-being at the time of their periods. But what most of them don't realise is that this need not be so. If they were to identify and remove the main offending substances from their diet or surroundings (preferably permanently but certainly on the 'at risk' days) these times would pass hardly noticed, instead of being dreaded, as they are by so many.

WHAT DISEASES?

As well as a wide range of patients, you will also notice a considerable range of diseases which responded to the approaches given in this book. Doctor Richard Mackarness, world-famous clinical ecologist and author of *Not all in the Mind* and *Chemical Victims*, reckons that over 50 per cent of all illnesses reported to the doctor have basis in allergy. One Merseyside GP trained in these principles thinks that this may be an underestimate in certain areas and that in his practice (a stressful urban district in an economically depressed area) it could be as high as 80 per cent. If you consider the list of symptoms which emerged in Dr Vicky Rippere's study quoted earlier in this chapter – and bear in mind that this is only part of a much longer list – you will see at once why these startling claims might be very close to the truth.

Chapter 3 gives an extended list of symptoms which frequently (not always) have an allergy base. You might like to glance ahead at it. You will see that by combining these symptoms in different ways it is possible to arrive at an almost infinite number of 'diseases' or states of illness. The majority of these syndromes would not coincide with any recognisable pathological process. Indeed, on investigating the condition in the conventional way, such as blood tests and X-rays, nothing can be found wrong. It is here that most doctors make a fatal flaw in reasoning. Since they cannot name what is wrong they assume it does not exist. This has been one of the problems. Because these states do not coincide with any identifiable disorders and since the patient's complaints often shift frequently from one symptom to another doctors usually consider these patients neurotic or inadequate in some way and thus the true nature of the illness is obscured.

The patient is told nothing is wrong, often in condemnatory or derisive tones and he or she is made to feel guilty or in some way at fault. They are told their illness is 'all in the mind' and stress is sometimes blamed. The sufferer usually gets a tranquilliser for 'nerves' which is easier for the doctor concerned and naturally suits the drugs companies, who will thus sell more of their goods. It could be argued that the boom in tranquillisers over the last three decades is nothing more than an index of the rise in environmental intolerance.

What is often ignored is that many of these sufferers are highly intelligent, capable and balanced people. They are often worried or alarmed about their condition but otherwise show no neurotic or unstable tendencies. Stress may be present but is really only making things worse, not the sole cause. These patients are often desperate to get well (and do so rapidly, given the right guidance). They want to lead busy and productive lives and it is cruel to assert that they are in some way creating their illness 'subconsciously'.

Of course, stress – any stress, mental or physical – will lower the body's resistance. Thus substances which it coped with, despite finding them hostile, are no longer tolerated and symptoms are often brought on by a stress crisis. To the lazy or casual observer it thus appears that the stress provoked the symptoms. Yet if the same individual were to remove from his diet and environment those factors which were hostile to him *he could then experience a great deal more stress than before, without any apparent ill effect at all.* Overworked executives and desperate housewives take note!

Incidentally, this line of logic applies also to other recognised triggers of symptoms, such as sunlight, damp weather, cold and exhaustion.

An explanation for the great variability of effects is given later under a discussion on target or shock organs. In the meantime, I give here a table grouping symptoms according to type or system and kindly supplied by Dr Michael Radcliffe from his own practice in Southampton. It is interesting to note that mental changes come highest on the list yet this is probably the most underdiagnosed group of allergy symptoms.

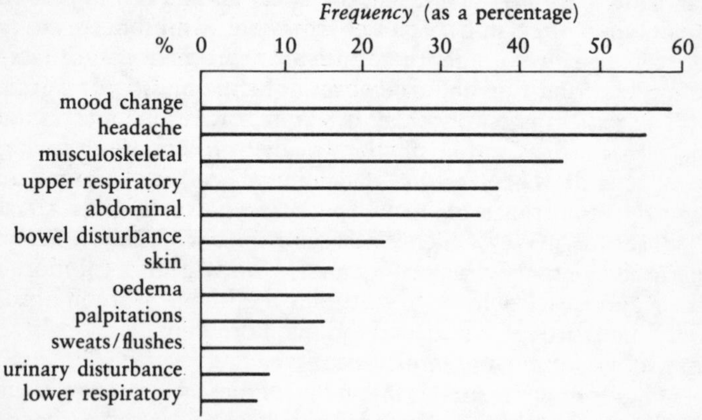

Fig. 1 *Percentage of patients with specific symptom relief in 100 polysymptomatic responders to dietary exclusion.*
(Reproduced here by permission of Dr Michael Radcliffe, General Practitioner, Clinical Teacher in Primary Medical Care, University of Southampton)

RECOGNISED DISEASES

In addition to the whole host of complaints to which no formal name can be given, a great many named diseases have also been shown to have an allergy basis. Some are no surprise: it has long been known that urticaria (hives) and asthma, for example, are such diseases. However, even in these conditions, it has not previously been recognised that food may play an important part. Everyone knows that asthmatics have problems with dust and feathers etc.; but tomatoes and wheat? Yet in my experience, better than 50 per cent of the trouble for asthmatics comes from diet and not from inhaled allergens. This is indeed fortunate because, whereas it may be hard to avoid dust, it isn't so difficult to give up eating certain foods.

Even more surprising, it has been discovered that many previously unsuspected diseases have a strong element of allergy. For example arthritis, migraine and peptic ulcer. Others include alcoholism, obesity, Crohn's disease (regional ileitis), colitis, depression, schizophrenia, vasculitis, paroxysmal tachycardia, cystitis (without evidence of infection), impotence, frigidity, premenstrual tension, Menière's disease, polymyositis and lupus erythematosus. There are others and it seems probable that the list may grow. This isn't to say that there is no other basis for these diseases; simply that many cases have been found to have an allergic element. Though some, for example Crohn's disease, are almost entirely allergic in origin.

In addition there are a number of borderline conditions where environmental factors (allergens) do seem to play a part on occasion. Multiple sclerosis is one and, taken early, the best results to date seem to come from the dietary approach. Psoriasis is another. Some cases respond easily. Others are so stubborn it raises the issue of whether or not there may or may not be more than one cause involved, perhaps several (this is aside from the hereditary or constitutional element and yet patients with a very convincing family history, making genetic factors seem all-important, may respond quickly and completely to the clinical ecology approach).

Unfortunately, conventional medicine seems to give little or no credence to the revolutionary ideas of the clinical ecologists, even though they themselves are medical doctors. Dietary improvements and changes in lifestyle are never considered as possible lines of treatment. Drugs and surgery always come first, drugs especially. At present this country spends a staggering sum on drugs each year. Yet many of these substances do more harm than good, and most are, at best, unnecessary.

Many patients have taken an interest in their complaints and asked questions of the specialists dealing with them (an audacity which, for some unaccountable reason, seems to send doctors rigidly on the defensive) such as 'Could my condition have anything to do with diet?' Almost invariably the answer is a categorical and uncompromising 'No', despite the fact that over 2,000 years ago Hippocrates wrote about the immutable relationship between diet and health. You and I might see sense in the cautious use of expressions such as 'maybe' or 'unlikely'.

I know of one NHS consultant physician, on a very large salary funded by the tax-payer, who declares openly 'I don't believe in diets'. One of his patients, who reported this to me, was understandably annoyed when his blood pressure (for which the said specialist was treating him) came down rapidly to normal, without the use of any drugs, on the Stone-Age Diet given later in this volume. Was this a coincidence? Read the rest of the evidence and then decide for yourself.

The unfortunate thing is that frequently the élite men and women of medicine are entirely immune to what the public at large thinks of them. They are all too often only concerned with the opinions of each other, which is a great pity. One can forgive a patient for feeling disillusioned if not openly contemptuous when, having been treated the conventional way for years with drugs causing unpleasant side-effects, he then gets better rapidly after a mere change in eating habits.

Considerations of this sort raise the question: Where are we going with modern medicine? Do we go further and further down the road of dangerous drugs, commando surgery, complex laboratory tests and ethereal diagnosis? Or is it time to sweep aside old dogmas and narrow 'scientific' thinking? The patient seems to have been lost sight of and, indeed, in some institutions one doubts that the system exists for his benefit so much as for the sake of scientific enquiry. Yet we should be listening to what he or she tells us not only about their condition but about factors which make it better or worse. After all, how he feels is his only criterion, not whether or not his sedimentation rate is back to normal.

Clinical ecology is a refreshing new science and as a discipline it seems truly to have come of age. Only just in the nick of time, one might add, in view of the rapid deterioration in the health of society at large due to environmental factors. As the old epidemic diseases come under control one by one, what is left is in the main diseases of deterioration in the optimum organism, in which I would tend to include cancer. We are well aware that extraneous factors play a major part in the causation of certain of these illnesses. What is being said by clinical ecologists is that it is something which will ultimately affect all of us. In that sense 'allergies', the subject of this book, concerns everyone and that is the theme I have taken.

VIRUS OR YEAST?

A startling possibility is that allergies may be precipitated by an infection of some kind. The two favourite theories at the moment are that the trouble may stem from either a virus infection (probably the Coxsackie strain) or a specific yeast *Candida albicans*, the organism which causes thrush.

Many allergy sufferers give a clear history of a virus-type illness. From it, they never really recovered their health and, years later, the illness is as bad as ever, with profound tiredness, weakness, pains, depression and other disabilities. Obviously the infection would have cleared up in that time. Furthermore, the on-going symptoms can often be shown to have an allergic basis, that is they will lift or ease after the principal dietary and environmental agents that make the individual feel unwell have been found and removed. Beyond these observations, the exact transition from an infective to an allergic disorder is simply not understood.

A number of names have been given to this distressing post-viral condition: myalgic encephalomyelitis, epidemic myasthenia, Iceland disease, Royal Free disease and post-viral fatigue syndrome are the principal ones. Since it has only been recognised in recent years, not enough investigation has been done to draw any general conclusions, except that there is clearly an organic basis for the condition. Drs P. O. Behan, W. M. H. Behan and E. J. Bell in Glasgow carried out extensive investigations in fifty such cases, which included five medical practitioners, eight nurses and a medical student! According to their report:

> All 50 cases had the same primary symptom, that of gross fatigue made worse by exercise. This fatigue was so conspicuous that one could see why the illness had been termed 'epidemic neuromyasthenia'. It was present at rest and quite different from that found in myasthenia or the myasthenic syndromes. The nearest clinical equivalent was the exhaustion reported by middle-aged males with multiple sclerosis affecting the spinal cord. The majority also complained of depression, difficulty in concentration, varying degrees of tinnitus, a feeling of disturbed equilibrium and hot and cold flushes. The illness was severe, with a high morbidity and a disastrous effect on their lives.[3]

Through extensive laboratory tests they were able to

demonstrate marked abnormalities in neuro-muscular transmission, muscle histological damage, reduced T-lympocyte activity (the ones involved in immunity) and other immunological changes. This puts paid to the usual theory that this condition is psychogenic in origin. Incidentally, you may be struck by the remarkable similarity between symptoms caused by this condition and those due to known allergic manifestations, listed in Chapter 3. It also bears repeating that most of these cases improve with the clinical ecology approach, identifying and removing allergens. This suggests that the fundamental damage is to the immune system (see Chapter 2).

It is highly probable that viral infections, even simple influenza, are potentially more damaging than was ever suspected previously. A clue is to be found in the work of Professor Lino Businco in Italy.[4] In a controlled experiment he subjected guinea pigs to daily inhalations of the influenza virus. After ten days of inhalation some of the animals were destroyed and examined; after twenty days a further number were killed and the final batch to be examined was killed after thirty days.

Not surprisingly, he found evidence of a lymphocyte response. But the extent of damage to major organs was a startling new discovery. The heart showed signs of atrophy and areas of degeneration; the kidneys were inflamed and showed a pattern not unlike chronic glomerulonephritis and the liver showed mild but diffuse fatty degeneration and concomitant fibroid reaction. Similarly the spleen, adrenal glands, thyroid, pancreas and testes were badly affected. Even the skin showed signs of atrophy of all structures and hair loss. Remember this was a controlled experiment, which is to say that there was a control group of animals not subjected to the virus inhalations. This control group remained normal and showed none of these changes.

The most significant changes were in the adrenal glands. These showed signs of haemorrhagic necrosis. Clearly their function was markedly affected and it is worthwhile recalling that the adrenal glands produce, among other substances, hormones which innervate the body at times of stress and enable it to cope. Thus a human being who suffered the same organ damage would become very intolerant of many simple substances, fatigued, depressed and very run down. You will see at once the connection between this wretched state and the general allergy syndrome which is described in this book. It is also possible that AIDS, which is now accepted as a viral disease, has some relevance here and you are referred to Appendix 4.

The second type of infection which has recently come under suspicion for causing allergies is fungal attack, especially, though by no means only, *Candida albicans*. This widespread mycobacterial agent, a kind of yeast also known as *Oidum* and *Monilia albicans*, is responsible for the disease known as thrush. It was known to Hippocrates and appeared frequently throughout the centuries in books relating to health, especially children's diseases, though it must be emphasised that it is by no means confined to children. Indeed it is considered that the normal source of infection is the mother; it lives in the female vagina as an almost 'routine' occurrence.

Under certain favourable conditions it may succeed in invading the body tissues and getting itself so entrenched in the cells that it overcomes normal immunity mechanisms and becomes virtually impossible to dislodge. This state is called Candidiasis or *Candida overgrowth* and goes far beyond what is normally meant by thrush. It seems to have its worst effect on the bowel where damage to the gut lining allows numerous toxic agents to pass through the wall into the blood and set up unpleasant symptoms which ordinarily would be kept in check by healthy bowel mucosa.

Pioneer work in this field was done by Dr Orian Truss, who first called attention to the symptoms created by *Candida*, *other than those of thrush itself*. These can be almost as wide as those due to allergies, and include depression, depersonalisation and other mental effects, digestive disturbances, food intolerance, muscle weakness, joint pains, sexual dysfunction and many others. Two of the most striking features of Candidiasis are the craving for sugar, which is of course fermented by the organism for food, and chemical intolerances.

This is basically a disease of malfunction and seems most readily to attack those whose health is already undermined by some other factors. The main predisposing circumstances can be summarized as follows:

1. any long-term debilitating illness;
2. oral contraceptives;
3. repeated or long-term use of antibiotics, especially the broad-spectrum types such as ampicillin and tetracycline;
4. use of corticosteroid drugs;

5. pregnancy;
6. twentieth-centry diets, rich in sugar and carbohydrates, poor in essential nutrients and minerals – a recipe for disaster.

Antibiotics are especially to blame. As Dr William Crook states they 'make yeasts grow like grass and weeds after a summer rainy spell'.[5] Yet the current fashion is to prescribe them with the abandon of handing out sweets to children. The least sign of an infection and the typical general practitioner is ready with a bottle or tablets of penicillin, often without precisely diagnosing the condition. Since over 70 per cent of sore throats are caused by viruses, which are unresponsive to antibiotics, it serves no purpose to prescribe them in the majority of cases. Similarly, millions of attacks of so-called cystitis are treated with broad-spectrum antibiotics, without any steps being taken to establish that there is a bacterial origin for the disease. Indeed, as you will read in this book, many cases are not infective at all, but caused by foods and chemicals having an irritant effect on the bladder. Thus even the label cystitis is a misnomer in some cases.

The end result of this massive overdosing with such drugs is not only that overgrowth of unpleasant micro-organisms is assisted but that resistant strains of bacteria are created. This has already begun to happen and will do so increasingly in future with frightening consequences. Our hospitals are now plagued with a type of resistant *staphylococcus* which cannot be treated with antibiotics. It simply cannot be harmed or destroyed and deaths from septicaemia due to this organism are steadily on the increase. In the end, unless this abuse ceases, we may find ourselves back in the era before penicillin, when we are once more helpless against bacteria and even a slight sore throat or a minor cut could be the passport to death.

To return to allergies, there is convincing evidence that hidden infections with *Candida* actually give rise to intolerance to foods. In other words, if the *Candida* infection is cleared up the patient feels better and is then able to tolerate well a number of substances which formerly caused problems. One of the worst effects of Candidiasis seems to be major chemical intolerance and this clears up quite nicely when the root cause is removed or controlled.

Nevertheless, few people can conquer this sort of problem purely by taking the drug Nystatin to kill off *Candida*. Some sort of environmental control programme will be required as well. This may be as simple as avoiding the most obvious food allergens or it may be as thorough as eliminating all badly tolerated foods, taking neutralising drops for others, adopting a rotation diet low in carbohydrate, taking vitamin and mineral supplements, and a complete house 'clean up' of chemicals. It depends obviously on the individual case. As Dr William Crook writes:

> During the past three years, I've treated over 400 patients with chronic health problems related to the 'yeast connection'. And although Nystatin and diet played an important role in helping most of these patients, many did not improve until other pieces of the puzzle were appropriately treated.[6]

An interesting curiosity connected with yeast infections is the disease with the Japanese name *meitei-sho* (drunk disease). It has been shown that in sufficient numbers these yeasts can ferment sugars in the bowel and release alcohol, a sort of on-the-spot distillery. Cases who became well and truly drunk without ever touching a drop of liquor have now been well documented. Studies of their bowel flora show overwhelming colonisation by *Candida* and other yeasts. It could hardly be called an allergy, as such, but certainly comes well within the purview of clinical ecologists. Look out for this condition in future. It will be with us while ever our diets are so loaded with sugars and carbohydrate and I expect to see it diagnosed more and more.

2

The Theory So Far

It must not be assumed that in this day and age of scientific discoveries we know a great deal about allergies. The fact is that we have very little understanding of this complex and mysterious phenomenon. There is even considerable dispute over what may be considered an allergy and what may not. Such controversies usually surround areas with no real concrete facts. As an example of this sort of thing, an argument raged for decades as to whether sunlight or vitamin D was required to treat rickets. Only the discovery that exposure to sunlight leads to the production of vitamin D in the skin put an end to the controversy and reconciled both points of view.

The word 'allergy' was coined in 1906 by von Pirquet, a Viennese physician. He described it as an acquired, specific, altered capacity to react to a physical substance on the part of the tissues of the body. This is an important first premise and worth considering in detail.

Acquired means that it is not in-born or constitutional, though there seems no longer any doubt that the tendency to develop reactions is familial. As far as our understanding extends at present, a substance must be encountered at least once before an allergy to it can be developed. (This is an important distinction from the 'low-grade poisoning' effect, discussed below.)

Babies may be born with an allergy but that does not seem to conflict with the above. It is believed that they may develop their allergy by contact with substances in the womb. Thus a rash present at birth may be due to milk (for example) in the mother's diet provoking an allergic reaction in her offspring via the placenta. Therefore it is still correct to use the term acquired.

Specific means that the reaction belongs only to that substance. Not all potential allergens cause trouble. Some people, it is true, are allergic to very many substances. But each reaction is unique *even though many of these reactions may produce the same effect.* To understand this it is necessary to be aware of the concept of the target or 'shock' organ. The resulting symptom from an allergic reaction, whatever it may be, depends on which part of the body bears the brunt of the attack. If the skin is affected a rash may result; if the lungs are mainly affected a wheeze or even an asthma attack could be caused; if the brain is affected, as it often is, any number of symptoms may result, as diverse as fatigue or inability to think clearly and depression or hallucination; there are many other possible effects, as you will read later. Yet the reaction to house dust is completely separate from the one for milk, even though both may have the same disastrous consequences. This is confirmed by the fact that it is possible to block one action independently of the other.

Altered means that the reaction is not 'normal', that is it is not shared by the remainder of the species. Pollen may make summer wretched for hay-fever sufferers. Yet it affects the rest of us not at all.

However, there is a grey area here. Some doctors report allergic reactions to substances such as phenol, petrol fumes and house gas. Small doses of the last, such as are to be found in the average home, may make certain individuals extremely ill. Yet the average person remains unaffected. If the concentration were higher, of course, we would all feel the effect. House gas is poisonous in sufficient concentration and would prove rapidly fatal to any one of us. Question: do we consider those who react to small concentrations to be experiencing unique allergy reactions, as described by von Pirquet; or is it simply that they poison more quickly than the rest of us? It may be right to consider this effect low-grade poisoning or even non-specific irritation instead, though many of my colleagues would not agree with this view. Not that it is a very important distinction, since in all cases it is best to avoid contact with the offending substance and the patient will feel better for doing so. In other words there is no practical outcome to the discussion.

Lastly, allergies are unquestionably *physical*. Stress may play a part in precipitating a crisis, and often does, but it is not the cause of the reaction. The fact that symptoms came on at a time of crisis may lead the physician to look no further than psychosomatic origins and thus the patient is denied the fruits of further enquiry. It is a pity because this 'all in the mind' diagnosis is rather condemnatory of the patient and often causes him or her to feel belittled and lose faith in the doctor. Moreover, this emphasis on the psychosomatic element is easy to refute by actual demonstration. If the physically harmful agents are removed from the patient's environment his or her tolerance of stress goes up enormously.

Thus stress is shown to be merely the trigger factor and not the root cause. It apparently lowers the patient's resistance, which is reduced to the point where agents which were quite well tolerated suddenly begin to have a marked adverse effect.

Therefore von Pirquet's definition is quite a good one. It is largely empirical and broad enough to encompass a number of possible mechanisms, even though he may not have intended this.

ANTIGENS AND ANTIBODIES

Subsequently a number of researchers entered the arena. It was discovered that certain defence mechanisms of the body were to blame in a number of allergy cases and attention was focused on this aspect of the disorder.

One of the most vital reactions that the body produces when 'invaded' by foreign substances is the manufacture of antibodies. These are chemicals which have a specific effect only on the foreign substance, to render it inert and easily dealt with. Examples of such alien stimulants are viruses and the toxins released by bacteria. These are known as antigens and stimulate the release of antibodies which are quite unique to themselves. These antibodies would cause inactivation of the virus, which could then be removed by available white blood cells. In the case of toxins, the antibody attaches to these and so alters them chemically, rendering them harmless. Thus the usefulness of this antigen-antibody reaction will be readily seen. It forms the basis of so-called immunity and is vital for the success of therapeutic vaccination.

To render someone safe from a disease such as polio, all that needs to be done is to introduce a few dead or inactive viruses into the body. These are recognised by their chemical characteristics and antibodies to the polio protein appear within a few days. Thus when live and disease-producing polio viruses enter the body, the antigen is already familar and antibodies to inactivate them can be produced immediately, to fight off the attack before the disease ever gets a hold. Indeed, without this facility, it is certain that we would not live long. Individuals born with a deficiency of this immunity system will soon die of even the most simple illness, such as the common sore throat. You may have seen these helpless creatures on television while awaiting bone-marrow transplants, living inside plastic tents, having to meet their friends and family through a barrier screen. They must be nursed in conditions of the strictest sterility. If they were to be exposed to everyday germs, such as your own body fights off every minute of the day, they would succumb helplessly in no time.

It makes no difference how your body meets micro-organisms and toxins, the result is the same. You may be deliberately immunised, using killed germs as described above, for diseases such as smallpox, cholera, whooping cough and diphtheria. Or you may contract an actual illness, suffer all the ill effects of it and then acquire natural immunity, to stop you getting it again. This is why it is rare to get a second attack of measles or mumps. After one dose, your body is ready next time around! (Incidentally the common cold is such a nuisance because the virus seems to keep changing all the time; as fast as you make antibodies they become ineffective against the new strain.)

What has this to do with allergies? Briefly, the body makes antibodies against things it shouldn't, for example dust or food. It treats them as 'intruders' in exactly the way it responds to micro-organisms, and attacks these substances furiously. The disturbance which ensues is what you recognise as a symptom, depending on which part of the body bears the brunt of the commotion. Allergic reactions of this type are therefore the result of a very useful defence mechanism going wrong and operating when we would rather it did not. We know this is the case in at least a proportion of allergic reactions, because the actual antibodies to milk, feathers, dust etc, can be identified in the blood.

HYPERSENSITIVITY

One thing that plagues medicine is its peculiar jargon. Most of it is derived from obscure Greek and Latin words, a throwback to the era of mediaeval alchemy and secret societies. For instance, no doctor would describe a patient's skin as red when he can use a juicy word such as erythematous, which means exactly the same thing.

Worse than that, there is a great deal of argument within the profession about what certain words mean. In fact I hope you will realise by reading this book that a lot of the so-called controversy about allergies doesn't really exist; it is largely a dispute about what should and should not be called by that term.

So it is with immune-reactions-gone-wrong as the cause of certain allergy reactions. The usual term now is hypersensitivity rather than allergy. The word supersensitivity was used as far back as von Pirquet's day but probably didn't sound quite obscure enough and so hypersensitivity is now preferred.

There are four basic mechanisms by which people react allergically and conventional physicians do not recognise allergy outside these disorders. They were originally classified by Coombs and Gell and are given below. However, the lay reader who finds the following section too technical should be able to skip it, without detracting from the value of the rest of the book. Interestingly, no part of these definitions refers to actual symptomatology. Laboratory tests only are used in detecting which mechanism is involved.

Type 1 reactions

Reaction resulting from the release of pharmacologically active substances such as histamine by certain cells such as mast cells after contact with specific antigens.

Ig-E (Immunoglobulin-E), a serum protein known to be associated with immediate-type allergic reactions, usually shows a significantly high titre in the blood.

The clinical conditions in which Type 1 reactions play a role include allergic extrinsic asthma, seasonal allergic rhinitis, systemic anaphylaxis, reactions to stinging insects, some reactions to food and drugs and some cases of urticaria.

The most usual test for Type 1 reactions is the intradermal prick test which is discussed in Chapter 5. Other tests include the radioallergosorbent test (RAST) and the passive transfer test based on the Prausnitz-Kustner reaction. They are explained in more detail in Chapter 6.

Type 2 reactions

Reactions which result when antibody reacts with antigenic components of a cell or with an antigen which has become intimately coupled with a cell or tissues.

The cells themselves become attacked and damaged by the antibodies. Occasionally this happens to the body's own tissues when we speak of auto-allergy or, more incorrectly perhaps, auto-immunity.

Diseases involving this type of process include certain haemolytic anaemias and purpuras (bruising disorder). This mechanism is also to blame for reactions to incompatible blood transfusions and may also play a part in multi-system hypersensitivity disorders such as systemic lupus or erythematosis (SLE).

Diagnosis is by detecting serum antibodies. A number of techniques exist which depend usually on the ability of serum to agglutinate cells (or even latex particles) previously treated with likely antigens.

The cytotoxic test referred to in Chapter 6 is probably dependent on Type 2 reactions.

Type 3 reactions

Type 3 reactions result from deposition of soluble antigen-antibody complexes, which are circulating in the blood, in tissues of the body. Inflammatory reactions surround these deposits and cause the disease process.

Examples of conditions in which Type 3 reactions play a part are serum sickness, rheumatoid arthritis, certain kidney disorders, SLE and the hypersensitivity reaction to lung aspergillosis.

Diagnosis is by detecting circulating immune complexes and by microscopy.

Type 4 reactions

This is often called the delayed hypersensitivity reaction, since typically it comes on after twelve to forty-eight hours, rather than at once. It appears to be due to sensitised white cells

(T-lymphocytes) attacking 'foreign' cells directly, rather than by means of antibodies.

Contact dermatitis is one disease caused by delayed hypersensitivity. Another is auto-immune thyroid disease. Perhaps some forms of drug sensitivity also and a few other medical curiosities.

Type 4 reactions are suspected whenever there is extensive involvement of lymphocytes in an inflammatory process. Confirmation can be by patch tests (see Chapter 5).

As Coombs and Gell point out:

> It must be stressed that the circumstances in which any of these four basic types of reaction may be studied in an uncomplicated form may be very special, and may, in fact, be seen only in certain animal species under quite strict experimental conditions. Again it must be emphasized that the pattern seen in any one human disease is often complex, involving not just one but several of the above pathways or responses.[1]

Type 1 reactions are often known as atopic reactions. Atopy (strange disease) is a word coined by Dr Arthur Coca in the USA, intended to cover all allergic manifestations, not just Type 1. He was a great figure in allergic medicine and managed to bridge the gap successfully between clinical ecology and immunology. He made significant contributions to both disciplines, though it must be said that he came in for a great deal of criticism from 'conventional' colleagues. He suggested another word 'idioblapsis' (life-spoiler) for non-immunological food allergies which has however lapsed into oblivion.

CLINICAL ECOLOGY

Unfortunately, during the 1920s, allergy reactions became increasingly identified with the antigen-antibody mechanisms described above. So much so that at present most doctors would be reluctant to diagnose an allergy without objective evidence of immunity to the substance involved. Dr Ben Feingold, elsewhere mentioned for his famous Feingold Diet, sums up this point of view thus:

> Allergy cannot be defined without a consideration of the nature of immunity. Immunity involves all the mechanisms concerned with the protection of the individual against the assault of foreign substances. A foreign substance is any material which the body does not

recognise as itself, ie. a part of itself . . . Since allergy is a variation of the basic immune mechanism, a discussion of allergy is actually a consideration of the mechanism of immunity.[2]

But some doctors were not content with this narrowing of purview. They saw in it an Alice in Wonderland sort of logic similar to stating that because some cats have long hair therefore only animals with long hair can be cats; this despite evidence before your very eyes that what you see is a short-haired cat!

Instead these doctors, mostly working in the USA, began to look for – and to find – unpleasant reactions to all sorts of physical substances as the cause of illness, purely on the basis that these substances appeared in real-life situations to make people ill *without any antibodies being present*. Food and chemical allergies were widespread, they claimed. One of them even stated, audaciously, that allergies would soon supersede germs as the number one cause of illness.

In fact this small but vociferous lobby of doctors protested loudly that we did not know what caused the majority of allergies but that the disordered immunity idea was far too simple and did not cover every possible mechanism. This hardly endeared them to the majority of their colleagues, who held views similar to Ben Feingold, quoted above.

With typical American flair for jazzy-sounding terminology, this group of doctors began to call themselves clinical ecologists. (*Ecology*: the study of an organism in relationship to its environment, from Greek *oikos*, house or home and *logos*, study).

Two separate disciplines eventually emerged, almost poles apart in their views. On the one hand were the conventional allergists, who laid great emphasis on careful objective testing and were highly scornful of any 'unscientific' approach. And on the other lay the clinical ecologists, who worked entirely empirically and considered subjective reports from the patient to be the best possible source of information in the tracking down of hostile influences and were equally dismissive of their allergy colleagues and their laboratory-oriented methodology which, they claimed, often had little real relevance to the patient's problems.

At the very root of the schism is continued argument about what should and shouldn't be covered by the term allergy. Perhaps the time has come to abandon the use of this contentious word altogether. *Intolerance* has been suggested as a possible alternative. Other offerings have been put forward but so far none has ousted the concept of 'allergy' in the public mind.

Theron Randolph, whose name you will encounter many times in any book on clinical ecology, suggested the terms exogeny and endogeny in medicine, which have not yet been accepted.[3] According to his view, exogeny is disease caused from without, i.e. environmentally. Endogeny, is disease from within. The first type of disorder postulates an individual who is potentially happy and healthy. The second type conceives only of sick people, rather like decrepit or malfunctioning machinery, who are basically unwell.

Modern medicine is endogenously oriented and its laboratory-based, reductionist, analytic, bodily-centred approach has come to dominate medicine almost entirely. That is until recently. Fortunately, there is the beginning of a swing in the opposite direction, towards a wider and more comprehensive view of health, which comes under the name of holistic medicine. Generally its methods are simple and inexpensive, relying very much on Mother Nature for the power to heal. Expensive drugs are shunned and so Big Business cannot get a foothold. Not surprisingly, therefore, the established system continues to be by far the most powerful lobby in officialdom, in hospitals and in medical education.

THE DIAGNOSTICO-THERAPEUTIC GAP

Unfortunately, the split between these two complementary views and the shift of emphasis entirely to endogeny occurred before the field of allergy and clinical ecology had developed fully. Indeed, this shift occurred before the full range of environmental excitants in the aetiology of disease had been identified or the more advanced systemic manifestations had been described. If this had not been so, it is quite probable that the endogenous approach would not have become so firmly entrenched, though this is to ignore, somewhat naively, the influence of vested interest.

Instead, we have what Randolph calls a diagnostico-therapeutic gap, that is a great indifference to the actual nature or causation of disease and instead an almost rigid fixation on studying how to treat its final end-result (symptoms). In grand rhetoric style, he is worth quoting more fully. Remember his medical career spans most of the clinical ecology versus allergy controversy we are referring to.

> It may be seen that interest in what was first described as allergy has taken two main and progressively polarized courses. The currently dominant one, best described as endogeny, consists principally of anthropocentrically focused [centred on the human organism] immunologic and other analytical approaches. Clinical manifestations are increasingly treated non-specifically and largely by means of drugs. The relative discontinuity between diagnosis and treatment in these circumstances constitutes what might be referred to as a diagnostico-therapeutic gap. Little serious effort is made to identify, measure, control, or neutralize etiologic environmental exposures or to determine the individual susceptibility of the host involved in such responses. As mentioned, this endogenous point of view, which emphasizes approaches to apparent bodily mechanisms, is relatively applicable en masse, and presently dominates teaching and research in this field, is best called clinical immunology.[4]

This polarisation has persisted to the present day though, as you will read by the end of this chapter, there is some sign of the gap being bridged by excellent studies carried out in the UK by competent and accredited specialists. The fact is that the time of clinical ecology is *now*. In our increasingly hostile world it is needed with considerable urgency and more and more people are seeking its aid and being glad they did. But like all new ideas, there is a period of acceptance. Hopefully this book and others like it will help to lessen the gestation period.

FOOD ALLERGIES, THE CINDERELLA ILLNESS

Notable among early clinical ecologists was Dr Albert Rowe from the USA. As early as the 1920s he began experimenting with elimination diets for the detection of food allergies. Fellow doctors ignored his findings completely because his investigations were not carried out in a 'scientific' manner. It is true that he did not carry out correctly controlled studies. But that hardly seems a reason to let such a possible momentous advance in the treatment of disease pass by unheeded.

There is in fact far too much emphasis in medicine on double-blind controlled trials. These may be very important when it comes to the use of drugs, most of which are potentially very damaging, but hardly relevant for simple matters such as the avoidance of certain foods and environmental chemicals. Besides, it bears emphasising that the drug Thalidomide, the story of which makes doctors and laymen alike shudder, passed all known and acceptable 'scientific' trials before being put to use.

Even today, most doctors have difficulty in accepting the idea of food allergies. Some of them are even openly derisive and opposed to the concept. In a recent, largely ignored, article in the *Lancet*, – a prestigious medical journal – two physicians, themselves committed to the belief that food allergy is a vital new discovery, were forced to play it low key and stated only modestly: 'Since many diseases are caused by the interaction of man with the environment, and since one of the major environmental factors is food, it seems feasible that dietary factors may cause disease.'[5]

Part of the problem is the extreme difficulty in demonstrating any immune-based reaction to foods. Most sensible people would wonder if this wasn't due to some shortcoming in the methods of testing, but the allergist (immunologist) takes this as proof-positive that food allergy is extremely rare and can be safely ignored. Nothing, it sometimes seems, will induce them to try the methods advocated by Albert Rowe and his followers. They are content to be guided by 'immunological principles soundly based on scientific facts' as one writer put it.

Lawrence Dickey, a well-known American ecologist and founder member of the American Society for Clinical Ecology, wrote scathingly about this:

> Food factors in disease, especially those of an allergic nature, are of great significance to those who have taken the trouble to become acquainted with the concepts and techniques of those who have devoted a great deal of time and energy to developing them. Unfortunately, this knowledge is not taught in medical schools.[6]

He also goes on to add as a barb, that conventional allergists have made 'no significant changes in either testing or specific antigen therapy since Noon and Freeman first described them in 1911'.

A WORKING DEFINITION

Clinical ecologists have not disputed the existence of the antigen-antibody mechanism in allergic disease. Rather they have tended to suggest that it isn't very important. What matters most in treating illness is what makes the patient well, not what brings greater comprehension to the physician.

They have evolved their own working definition of what an allergy is. Roughly speaking they consider an allergy to be present if:

1. avoiding the suspected allergen is shown to result in clinical improvement;
2. re-exposure to it leads to clinical worsening;
3. no other obvious cause is found.

However, there are certain 'catches' to this definition, as you will learn later. A patient may not necessarily feel better avoiding an allergen, if exposure to several others remains unchecked. Also, a true allergen may not cause a reaction when eaten (for example) if the interval since last taking the food is less than about five days. This is due to what is called the masking effect and appears to apply equally to chemical and other allergens, not just to food. The phenomenon is explained in more detail under hidden allergies below.

So to be completely scientific about this we should say that if avoiding a substance leads to improvement and then re-exposure to it causes symptoms, then it is definitely an allergen (as far as a clinical ecologist is concerned). If neither holds true then it may or may not be an allergen. In other words, failure to meet the three requirements above is not proof of non-allergenicity, *unless certain criteria are strictly observed*. It is unfamiliarity with these criteria that leads the uninformed observer to dispute the existence of a true allergy. The full test procedure for food is described in Chapter 5.

THE HIDDEN ALLERGY

One of the dividing principles between allergy and clinical ecology is the concept of the hidden or masked allergy. Conventional allergists don't recognise the existence of the phenomenon. Clinical ecologists use an understanding of it all the time, to be able to treat many patients and many diseases.

Dr E. C. Hamlyn, a doctor from Ivybridge in Devon, sums up some of the main characteristics of the hidden (masked) allergy quite elegantly:

> A postulated mechanism of illness. Emprirical evidence from clinical

experience suggests that a broad spectrum of common ailments is caused by muted allergy. Muting is caused by frequent exposure. By a process of adaptation this response becomes masked and cause and effect is obscured.

CAUSES.

Pollution of the environment is implicated.

1. The onset of this type of illness often follows an incident of pollution.
2. These illnesses are rare prior to pollution.
3. These illnesses tend to abate if pollution is reduced.
4. Once acquired these illnesses often become familial.
5. Increasing environmental pollution coupled to the phenomenon of acquired heredity explains the enormous increase in allergic disorders.

Forms of pollution:

a. Intentional additives to foodstuffs and water. eg. colouring, preservatives, flavourings, fluoride.
b. Vitiation of foodstuffs. eg. hybrids, processing of foods, synthetic foods.
c. Pollution by commercial 'necessity' eg. pesticides and herbicides. Hormones and antibiotics. Lead from petrol.
d. Pollution by industrial negligence. eg. radio-active waste pumped into the Irish Sea. Industrial effluent discharged into lakes and rivers. Products of combustion released into the atmosphere.
e. Abuse of drugs by patient and doctor alike.
f. Occupational exposure to chemicals.

PATHOLOGY.

Little is known.

SYMPTOMS.

Symptoms are Protean, Perverse, Bizarre, Changeable and Paradoxical.

Protean. The foremost characteristic of illness due to masked allergy is the incredibility of variation in symptomatology.

Perverse. Perversion of perception is a prime ingredient of this form of illness and constantly endangers its credibility. A superacuity of taste smell or hearing are examples.

Bizarre. Symptoms tend to bear no relationship to anatomical structure, to be quite unique to the individual and to defy description in ordinary terms, e.g. a feeling of cobwebs over the face, legs full of boiling water, a feeling as though floating outside the body, etc.

Changeable. Symptoms come and go without apparent reason. Symptoms change from time to time, moving from one system to another, e.g. eczema, asthma, migraine, spastic colon, peptic ulcer...

Paradoxical. These are illnesses full of contradiction. Lethargy that swings in and out of hyperactivity, anorexia with bouts of food bingeing, miserably cold or tormented by heat, tachycardia (fast heart) alternating with pseudo-heart block.

There are five characteristics of masked allergy which obscure the diagnosis.

1. The patient tends to become addicted to the food to which he is allergic.
2. He gets ill if he stops eating the offending food.
3. He feels better when he resumes eating that food.
4. Withdrawal symptoms may last for several days.
5. When he resumes eating the offending food after the withdrawal symptoms have gone, there may be an immediate reaction, a long delayed reaction or no reaction at all.[7]

So you will see, from this brief synopsis, that we are dealing with a phenomenon which is both complex and mysterious. No wonder recognition has been so long in coming!

A good illustrative case is that of Dr Herbert Rinkel, one of the founders of the science of clinical ecology. As so often happens in the evolution of knowledge, a chance observation made by the right person, someone with enough skill and presence of mind to comprehend the significance of what happened, led to a major discovery.

Rinkel suffered greatly from catarrh. This was at a time when he was studying medicine as a mature student. Naturally, this was a difficult period for him financially. To help out, his father regularly sent crates of eggs from the family farm in Kansas. Rinkel coped but inexplicably he became more and more ill as time went by.

Years later, Rinkel noticed that eating several eggs at once made him feel very ill. So he tried the experiment of eliminating eggs from his diet altogether. This was the first time he had ever gone without eggs and he was gratified to find that he felt much better. But then a few days later, as the story goes, he ate a cake with eggs in it quite by mistake and passed out.

He realised that he was allergic to eggs but what intrigued him more was the fact that he had eaten them for years without realising! He reasoned that the frequent exposures to egg had caused the reaction to obscure itself. Yet there was no doubt it was a severe reaction: it actually made him unconscious!

What seems to happen is that the body is able to resist the worst effects of a frequently encountered allergen, at least part of the time. Only when too much is encountered do symptoms break through. This also seems to happen when the body's resistance is lowered temporarily, such as due to stress or acute illness. Many people are able to date the onset of their illness by the incidence of some unfortunate stress in life. To understand more about why masked allergies should behave in this way it is necessary to jump forward some years, to 1956 to be exact, and the publication by Hans Selye of his book *The Stress of Life* and its description of the General Adaptation Syndrome.

THE GENERAL ADAPTATION SYNDROME (GAS for short)

Selye noticed that organisms under stress exhibit three well-defined stages of response to that stress. This is as true for rats subject to constant harassment as for human beings undergoing repeated traumas or minor infections.

First the organism or individual is stimulated by the stress, finds it unpleasant and takes necessary avoiding action if possible. Symptoms will certainly be noticed but these cease as soon as exposure to the stress stops. This is stage one.

In the second stage, if the assault continues, the organism or individual learns to cope with the stress and ignores it. Apparently little ill-effect is noticed. This may be called *adaptation*, a term which the clinical ecologists have certainly taken to themselves.

However, even though no apparent adverse effects are noticed, the resistance of the tissues of the body may be being constantly eroded. While all appears quiet, there is nevertheless a battle going on and sooner or later there has to be a winner and a loser. Thus eventually the body's resistance is completely exhausted and the stress can no longer be coped with. Symptoms then return and often do so much more severely, for now the organism or individual has little power of recovery left.

Selye called these stages the General Adaptation Syndrome, since the theory seems to be so widely applicable (all good hypotheses are simple and yet explain a wide variety of effects).

It is only a theory at this stage but a very plausible one indeed. It is certainly attractive to clinical ecologists, as it seems to explain so well what happens during the history of a person's allergies.

Take an example of allergy to milk to illustrate the principle. A child may be made quite ill with milk. Perhaps no-one notices, or they do but assume they must be mistaken, because they have heard that milk is good for us and that children need large quantities of it (both of which are common misconceptions about milk!). The parents, who are trying to do their best for the child, insist that he drink his milk regularly. He gets lots of colds and sore throats and cries miserably but that is considered 'normal' for a child in this day and age. Milk, the real culprit, goes undetected. This is stage 1 of adaptation (the child is unadapted, clearly).

But the parents persist and eventually milk no longer makes the child ill. They feel vindicated and assume that the 'allergy', if they ever believed in it, has cleared up. All is now well, they think, and attach no significance to the occasional bouts of illness suffered by the child, or that he is 'moody' and seems inattentive at school. This is stage two and the child may be said to be adapted to milk.

But then, in later life, the child who is now an adult suffers with migraines and severe indigestion. He goes to the doctor and is prescribed pain killers, which make his stomach worse and he gets a peptic ulcer, said to be due to the overuse of pain killers. If he is really unlucky, he may have an acute episode and be rushed to hospital. There, the chances are, he will be supplied with plentiful milk, since that is known frequently to have a soothing effect on ulcers. Yet all the time, no-one suspects the real reason he is ill. He is now in stage three, *maladapted* to milk and, unless a clinical ecologist or a knowledgeable aunty who has heard of milk allergy rescues him, he is likely to remain very ill indeed for the rest of his life. Perhaps he will have occasional trouble-free bouts but the general trend will be downwards.

Thus parents should never force their children to eat food which they don't seem to like. It might be an instinctive aversion due to an allergy.

Interestingly, that same patient might have become actually addicted to milk. He may have come to consume large quantities of milk and, in the later stages of his illness, he may have noticed that it made him 'feel better'. If he avoided it he would feel grumpy and under the weather and his next milk feed would remedy this. He might even have believed that milk was good for him. Hadn't his mother always said so!

This is addiction, real addiction in medical terms and is one of the characteristics of later stage 2 and stage 3 maladaptation to food and other allergies. In the table of symptoms given in Chapter 3 you will see listed symptoms such as 'crabby on waking', 'slow getting started in the morning' and so on. These feelings, though admittedly very common, are nevertheless almost diagnostic of food allergy. What happens is that, by breakfast time, the person has been off food for twelve to fourteen hours and is beginning to get *withdrawal symptoms*, in exactly the same way that an alcoholic does when he comes off the bottle. The day's first cup of tea and bread or cereal give that 'fix' which is so essential to the drug addict and the withdrawal effects clear – until the next morning.

There is no difference in character between this type of addiction and that due to drugs. It is merely more acceptable socially. Moreover, the withdrawal symptoms from food exclusion diets, such as described in Chapter 4 can, in exceptional cases, be just as severe as with heroin.

Really, maladaptation to a food (or chemical or other substance) is the same as a hidden allergy. Provided the individual eats or drinks that food several times a week, it is permanently inside him and keeps the withdrawal effects at bay. Frequent encounters obscure the symptoms, hence the alternative name of masked allergy, as described by Ted Hamlyn above.

Addiction is thus a valuable clue to food allergies. Favourite or binged items in the diet come under immediate heavy suspicion from a clinical ecologist who knows what to look for. It could be said, with somewhat wry humour and not a little truth, that if every sick individual were told simply to give up all their favourite foods many of them would recover rapidly.

You will see now why it is not necessarily immediately true that if an allergic patient avoids his allergen he may feel better. For a time he may have symptoms which are worse! Also, he may *not* be made ill by returning to that food within five days, because his body will not be cleared of it and the masking effect may prevent any apparent ill effect whatever. This explains the strict protocol for testing a food outlined in Chapter 4.

CHEMICAL ALLERGIES

Great emphasis is laid by clinical ecologists on foods as the subject of hidden allergies. Rightly so, as they are by far the most common cause. However, they are not the only allergens encountered as the early workers, with acumen unhindered by personal prejudices, were soon to discover. Dust, feathers and danders (skin scales, such as dandruff) as allergens have, of course, been known for a long time. But it soon became clear that chemicals too can cause problems.

We have been doing more and more to pollute our environment since the Industrial Revolution and, inevitably it seems, the penalty must be paid until we come to our senses and put a stop to widespread contamination of the world we live in. The fact is, that despite assurances by government watchdogs who should know better, and the arrogant indifference of huge industrial conglomerates who are to blame, there is abundant evidence that this pollution is harmful to human (and other) life.

Is pollution new? I am often asked why it is that allergic disease seems to be on the increase and it is easy to point glibly to pollution and say there is your answer. Every now and then someone who is quick-witted points out that pollution has been around for over a century and yet allergies seem to have grown so enormously in only the last two or three decades.

True. In Victoria's reign in English towns, there must have been even worse pollution than today. They had gas (a potent hydrocarbon allergen), steam engines billowing smoke, unrestricted effluvia from burgeoning factories dealing in chemicals and, perhaps worst of all, countless coal-burning home fires. The last, as well as soot, give off oxides of sulphur which cause the so-called acid rain that is harsh enough literally to dissolve our city buildings, never mind harm humans. It is the sulphur dioxide that makes smog such a deadly killer to the old and infirm.

With new regulations enforcing smokeless zones in our cities this atmospheric pollution in towns is now far less than it was just after the last war. Buildings which are stripped and washed now stay clean, a testimony to the effectiveness of this environmental campaign. Smog, as such, is now largely a thing of the past here. Yet if you visit even a modest English village in winter, where open coal fires are still allowed, you will notice a distinct smoke pall except when breezes are fresh, a sorry reminder of what things must once have been like. Our city air is thus arguably cleaner than it was last century and opponents of the theory are quite right to point this out.

However, there are several reasons which would still explain why we are more polluted chemically in the present day. Firstly, we have the motor car, which gives off toxic fumes. Enough, indeed, in cities such as Los Angeles to cause 'auto-exhaust smog' due to the sheer numbers of cars present. Secondly, we have much more home pollution, such as powerful detergents, deodorants, solvents and that most obnoxious of toxins, the aerosol spray can. It is the propellent itself, a fluorinated hydrocarbon, which is such a potent poison, regardless of whether the spray is a furniture polish, hair spray, deodorant or whatever. Lastly, and I believe the most important of all, we have had in recent decades the almost indiscriminate use of powerful biocidal chemicals, especially in agriculture. On an unprecedented scale we have been smothering our foods in deadly fungicides, weed-killers and pesticides. These substances are still present on eating, despite cooking and processing, and are dangerous and extremely hostile to life. It is folly in the extreme to imagine that what kills beetles, bugs and fungi won't also harm us, given enough quantity. The problem is: how much is enough to be harmful?

The simple answer is that nobody knows. Glib assurances by government scientists or, even more suspect, the chemical manufacturing companies' own chemists, must be viewed as what they are – deliberate attempts to mislead the public into a false sense of security. No scientist of integrity would for a second presume that he knew anything about the complex interactions of these chemicals. Studies using animals exposed to such chemicals singly give us no clue as to the effects in actual use. But from the behaviour of other substances, such as drugs acting together, we can be fairly certain that poisons potentiate each other. That is, their effect together is far worse than the summation of individual toxic effects.

What the boffins don't seem to want to take into their calculations is the fact that a dose which may possibly be safe for the majority of people, will certainly make *some* of us ill. There is a certain biological principle involved here, best considered under the 'biological distribution curve' (often called a cocked-hat curve from its invariable shape). An example is shown below, in relation to height of adult males. The horizontal axis gives the height parameter and the upright axis gives the numbers of individuals with that exact height characteristic. As you can see the majority of males are bunched at around 5 feet 9 inches, which is average. But there is a steadily decreasing number who vary from this upwards or downwards, fewer and fewer the further from average the height in question. Quite a lot of people are over 6 feet, for example. A lot fewer are over 6 feet 6 inches. Only a tiny proportion exceed 7 feet.

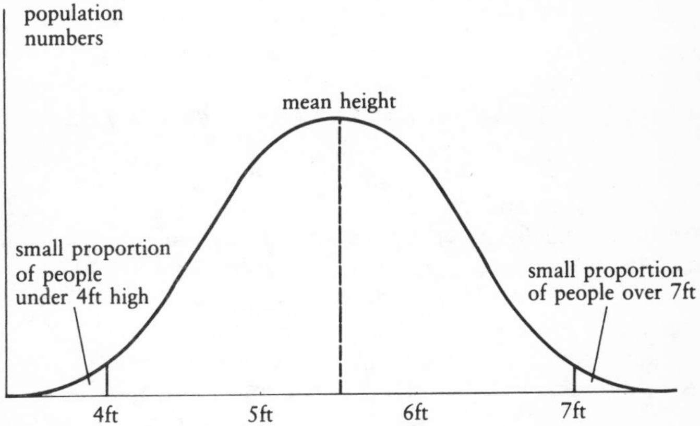

Fig. 2 *Height distribution curve*

The interesting point about this type of curve is that it has wide applicability in studying life forms. For instance it would apply straightforwardly to the way in which the toxic effects of a given poison varied according to dose. In other words, the majority of people would be made ill by a similar dose. But some would tolerate enormous doses and still not feel any real effect. Rather more problematical, the left hand end of that curve represents a small proportion of individuals who will be made severely ill by even a tiny dose. They too are part of the biological normal range.

The question is: do we set toxic levels that are safe for the majority or do we make sure that no one at all feels ill with a permitted dose? Bear in mind also that this is over simple in that toxic effects are complicated when more than one substance is

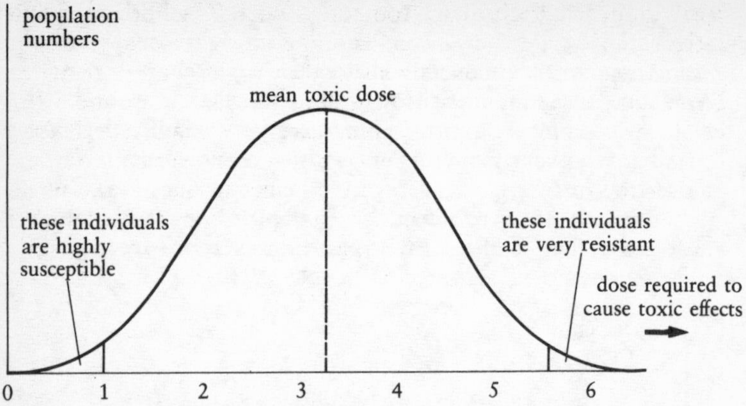

Fig. 3 *Distribution curve applied to chemical toxicity*

present at the same time. I think you will agree it is a vexed question. I would like to think that, in a just and compassionate society, everyone is protected. It isn't enough just to dismiss those at the bottom of the ladder as freaks and say hard luck to them.

Of course, there are other factors to take into account, such as economics. Food production is about starving millions and we are right to do what we can to increase productivity. But the irony of it is that those countries who are responsible for the chemical pollution on the whole produce food far in excess of their needs, which doesn't appear to benefit countries on the starvation line. Thus it isn't easy to justify the use of chemicals to increase productivity when the end-result is only more profits for some and not better human welfare.

A very capable but, frankly, depressing book on this topic is *Silent Spring* by Rachel Carson. She outlines numerous disasters due to potent herbicides, insecticides, etc. used in 'modern' farming, and cites ample evidence of their extremely toxic effects on man and beast. Her book was written in the early 1960s yet how much worse today are the problems she was warning us about. These agricultural chemicals are, I believe, the prime offenders when we speak of present-day pollution and the main difference factor in the dramatic rise in allergic or maladaptive disease. It is a real rise, incidentally, not simply that it is being diagnosed more often (though that, too, is a further reason for the increase).

In Britain today practically all food crops are being sprayed. From figures produced by the Ministry in the 1970s, 99 per cent of all cereals, 98 per cent of potatoes, beet and beans, 92 per cent of orchard crops and 94 per cent of vegetables were sprayed at least once and in most cases many times.

Unfortunately, the problem doesn't just confine itself to those chemicals ingested in food. Because of very wasteful spraying procedures (which manufacturers encourage, since they sell more chemical), 20 per cent or more of the spray substances, droplet particles of under 100 microns, remain indefinitely in the atmosphere. These are not heavy enough to fall. Conservative estimates put the total quantity of chemical-containing mixtures sprayed on crops at about one billion gallons; that means some 200 million gallons each year are going into the air we breathe. Britain, of course, has a substantial contribution to this pall of poison. Could there be any truth in the Norwegians' claim that the air from Britain is damaging their trees?

In the UK the agricultural chemical industry is not subject to any restrictions. There are no controls or checks. All that exists is the Pesticide Safety Precaution Scheme which is regulated by the industry itself using only data supplied by manufacturers, itself bent on fat profits and not human health. Often this information is surrounded by a wall of secrecy, under the guise of commercial confidentiality, while in fact it effectively denies public scrutiny by unbiased workers who could look after the interests of you and me. Concerned? You'd better be. It is rather like asking for the police force to be taken over by established criminals. The results would be predictably poor for law and order.

Nor should your anxiety rest there. Legislation has been mooted which would enshrine the PSPS instructions in law. As the Soil Association point out in their booklet *Pall of Poison*,

> In practise this means that chemical companies themselves will decide what instructions for use go on chemical product labels and how much chemical the farmer *has* to apply. All the indications are that these will be based on conventional spray usage. Farmers who are currently breaking the PSPS regulations by applying *less* chemicals may soon be breaking the law. The new legislation now being prepared could be an excuse for the chemical industry to hold

> up and make illegal progress towards safer, much reduced spraying and maintain profits in the excess – all under the banner of pollution control.[8]

It's the most outrageous case of Big Business hijacking the vehicle of democracy for the purpose of extorting money corruptly ever to come before our parliament.

And what is the Ministry of Agriculture and Fisheries doing about it? Nothing. Despite the strident cries of highly informed individuals, who clearly have no financial interest in the matter, the worthies of Whitehall are doing not a thing.

The official view is that all these chemicals are safe. We are told that provided the instructions are followed nothing could possibly go wrong. Yet it has been demonstrated that much of the data on safety tests was forged deliberately (the IBT scandal), no long term tests have been carried out, nobody knows what 'safe' levels are and so instructions are meaningless guidelines and, last but not least, who is to say that the instructions *are* applied? Nobody exists to check up on the farmer or chemicals salesman.

Official reassurances? Poof!

LOW-GRADE POISONING

After that political and philosophical departure, we return to clinical ecology. The first work setting down clearly the ill-effects of chemicals was *Human Ecology and Susceptibility to the Chemical Environment* by Dr Theron Randolph in 1962. From that date clinical ecology can be said to have arrived. This classic revelatory book should be required reading for all medical students before graduating as doctors and yet, sad to say, very few medical practitioners have even heard of it or are familiar with the important clinical data it propounds.

It is a sad commentary on our profession that, for all his advanced and enlightened work, Randolph had to endure years of scorn from his colleagues. Even now, doyen among clinical ecologists who hold him in great regard, he is barely recognised as the great teacher he is. To delve into its pages was to me, a practising physician, a journey of discovery and surprise. Here for the first time were extraordinary cases of people made ill by petrol fumes, aerosols, gloss paint, carpets, detergents, household gas, plastics, waxes, metal polish ... substances which don't bother the average individual and so had hitherto been ignored.

Unfortunately his published accounts, largely anecdotal, did not conform to accepted scientific standards for 'proof'. Nevertheless, the discoveries he sets out are easy to verify if any doctor cares to take the trouble to try them for himself. It is a pity that so many modern doctors will not make judgements for themselves but prefer to let others do the work and are only prepared to believe an observation if it has been reported in one or other of the prestigious journals given over for the purpose.

THE LAST TWO DECADES

From the sixties onwards, clinical ecology started to move apace. In 1965 a group of doctors in the USA, among them Theron Randolph, Herbert Rinkel, Arthur Coca, Warren T. Vaughan and Harris Hosen, founded the Society for Clinical Ecology, which began to make its voice felt everywhere except, unfortunately, where it counted most – medical schools, where clinical ecology should be put on the curricula. Nevertheless, it has done a great deal to educate doctors who are willing to listen and learn, running regular seminars to explain the methodology to practitioners who want to give it a try.

In the UK in the late seventies a similar group of doctors founded what was at first known as the Clinical Ecology Group. Richard Mackarness was a key figure in its inception. Then in 1983 we changed the name to the British Society for Clinical Ecology. In 1985 yet another change was mooted, it being felt that clinical ecology still didn't have a sufficiently comprehensive meaning and it seems likely that the word allergy will feature very prominently in the new name. Thus we are finally 'coming out' as the homosexuals say and tackling the old controversy about terminology head on.

Richard Mackarness, a GP turned psychiatrist, turned clinical ecologist, was by this time famous the world over. His best-selling book *Not All in the Mind* (and later its successor *Chemical Victims)*, together with numerous broadcasts – including a one-hour television documentary – did a great deal to popularise the subject of allergies, especially those relating to foods. He was widely respected and admired by clinical ecologists both sides of the Atlantic and indeed continues to be, despite his retirement. He made a number of contributions to the science, notable among which was the Stone-Age Diet (see Chapter 4) which he so named because archeological evidence suggests it was Man's natural diet.

Mackarness was responsible, along with Mrs Amelia Nathan-Hill, one of his patients, for setting up an information body called Action Against Allergy, which is a registered British charity. It does a great deal to promote further understanding of both the medical and sociological aspects of allergy disease. It has an excellent lending library facility for doctors, which aims to try and keep abreast of current developments.

It is probably no exaggeration to say that due to the Mackarness books and the work of Action Against Allergy public consciousness of the problem has for years been way ahead of interest by the medical profession. This is reflected in the fact that AAA gets thousands of letters from depressed and helpless patients who feel that allergy is very much the cause of their problem and yet their own doctor won't help, often being positively opposed to the idea of the existence of such a phenomenon as food and chemical allergies.

However, times are changing. The biggest single factor in the opposition from doctors as a group has been the lack of so-called scientific proof of the existence of food and other allergies. (When I meet this argument I like to point out that gravity has never been *proven*. We merely surmise it to exist because it explains many facts that can be directly observed!)

The fact is that many good papers have been prepared by clinical ecologists, following all accepted criteria *and no reputable journal would publish them*. The reason is not hard to find: all medical periodicals rely heavily on advertising revenues to pay their way. These come almost exclusively from drug companies who would lose huge incomes if the clinical ecologists had their way! So much for the contention that it is unscientific. So much also for the integrity of much of the criticism of this work.

In Britain, things are a little less cynical. Here, at last, satisfactory studies are being carried out, and really the results are very hard to argue with. Traditionally, the British have always been very good at this sort of thing. So whereas clinical ecology was quite definitely spawned in the USA, it remains to us to rear the offspring.

First among these was a largely forgotten paper published in the *Lancet* in 1978. Briefly it concerned a double-blind study using induction via a naso-gastric tube. In other words neither the patient nor the clinicians had any knowledge of what was being administered, so preconceptions could not interfere with the true findings. Yet there was a remarkable correlation between foods presumed allergenic and the causation of symptoms. Nevertheless, in those days it was considered such a shocking and revolutionary idea that the authors felt able to make only the cautious statement: 'This clinical study supports the view that some foods may cause widespread and disabling symptoms in people who are sensitive to them.'[9]

In 1982, a group of workers at Cambridge studied twenty-one patients with irritable bowel syndrome by means of diet restructuring. Each began with a week eating only one fruit and one meat of his or her choice. Those whose symptoms remitted were then tested by reintroducing single foods double blind through a naso-gastric tube (that is to say, in this study also, with neither the patient nor the attendant knowing what the food was) and noting the reactions. Fourteen patients cleared their symptoms on the first stage of the diet. (A clinical ecologist would assume that those who did not recover were allergic to one or other of the permitted foods and try to find another combination.) On carrying out the challenges the following foods were found to provoke reactions: wheat (nine patients), corn (five), dairy products (four), coffee (four), tea (three) and citrus fruits (two). Naturally, some patients were sensitive to more than one food.[10]

Clinical ecologists have been saying for years that this condition is due to food and chemical allergy. But the value of this study is that it was carried out in accordance with accepted investigatory practice and thus the findings are hard to argue with. Nevertheless, sceptics are abundant.

Probably the most significant study to date was carried out on children who were patients at the Hospital for Sick Children and Institute of Child Health, Great Ormond Street, London. The findings are given here in summary:

> 93% of 88 children with severe frequent migraine recovered on oligoantigenic diets; the causative foods were found by sequential reintroduction, and the role of foods provoking migraine was

> established by a double-blind controlled trial of 40 of the children. Most patients responded to several foods. Many foods were involved, suggesting an allergic rather than an idiosyncratic (metabolic) pathogenesis. Associated symptoms which improved in addition to the headache included abdominal pain, behaviour disorder, fits, asthma and eczema. In most of the patients in whom migraine was provoked by non-specific factors, such as blows to the head, exercise, and flashing lights, this provocation no longer occurred while they were on the diet.[11]

So much for doctors who say there is no such thing as food allergy. Oligoantigenic, by the way, means low in likely allergens (antigens). The importance of this study is that it meets the most rigorous standards of scientific 'proof' and the doctors involved, under Professor Soothill, are competent 'no nonsense' workers. I can only say that clinical ecologists, most of whom themselves run small individual clinics and have no funds available for such extensive research, look forward to the publication of more such papers. It is hard for them not to take the 'I told you so' stand.

There is an unfortunate tendency for Dr Hunter and Professor Soothill to talk as if they had personally discovered clinical ecology phenomena. In their own minds they perhaps did, since they themselves were part of the sceptical establishment until they took the trouble to investigate matters for themselves. But I would like to hear them give a little more credit to Albert Rowe, Herbert Rinkel and Theron Randolph, who made the discoveries decades ago. Nevertheless, clinical ecologists point to their work with great satisfaction and we are grateful for these tools to use on our rigidly orthodox colleagues, even if it is only a case of sticks to beat the lazy and feeble-minded.

A more recent and, frankly, less useful publication came in 1984 with the report on food intolerance and food aversion by the Royal College of General Practitioners and the British Nutrition Foundation. It stands, to re-use Lawrence Dickey's wonderful phrase, as a major contribution to ignorance on this topic. It was briefed to review evidence for the phenomenon of food allergy yet the way in which it did this could only be described as partial and biased, seeming to ignore the evidence which didn't fit the preconceived ideas of the creators. The title carefully avoids the term allergy and, as you may surmise, this is reserved only for the immunologically proved manifestation of food allergy and so effectively consigns to the rubbish bin the opinions of clinical ecologists all over the world.

As an example of this absurd slanting, the report accepts the Professor Soothill's Great Ormond Street double-blind study evidence for migraine in children (and incidentally then says there is no evidence that food causes migraine in adults). The report goes on to claim that there is no evidence that hyperactivity in children is caused by diet. Yet Professor Soothill's group stated quite clearly that among a number of unlooked for improvements among the migraine children was the fact that thirty-six out of forty-one hyperactive children recovered completely and returned to normal behaviour. This is clearly a case of ignoring unwanted facts.

Another glaring instance of finding what you want to find is the quotation of statistics to support the efficacy of the skin prick test and the RAST test for serum IgE (see chapters 5 and 6 for an explanation of these tests). The report says that both these tests 'have been claimed to correlate well with clinical evidence of food allergy'.

In fact Soothill's study, which was accepted by the committee remember, states quite clearly that

> Though some prick tests for foods which caused symptoms were positive the association was not strong and *only 3 patients would have recovered if they had avoided only foods to which they had positive prick tests*. Similarly 28% of the 64 patients had high serum IgE levels, but IgE antibodies were not helpful in identifying causative foods.[12]

(My italics, K. M.) Can anyone defend this report as helpful guidance for the uninformed?

The fact is that the committee, under Professor Maurice Lessof, see themselves as belonging to the traditionalists, with their heads firmly buried in immunological sand and don't want to admit the validity of clinical ecology and its methods. Perhaps they feel threatened as clinical ecologists are unreservedly critical of the dangers of their kind of scientific medicine and constantly harp on on the fact that it poses risks to the patient and often causes effects which are as bad or worse than the original disease process.

I hope now, at the end of this chapter, you realise that there are two distinct schools of thought on allergy and that should your doctor suggest you visit an allergy 'specialist' you find out if he is an immunologically oriented one. If so you may expect no more than a few tests and probably being told that you have 'no allergies', despite being ill. The chances are no other explanation will be offered as to the origin of your complaint, yet do not be surprised if you are given drugs, even in the absence of a clear-cut diagnosis.

Perhaps you should insist on seeing a clinical ecologist instead (who, as you will by now know, misdefines and misuses all his words!) as he is certainly unlikely to give up experimenting with diets and environmental tests until he has found *what is making you ill*.

Even then, there are good and bad clinical ecologists. The point to look for is does he or she expect you to take an active participation in your illness? Being given endless neutralising drops (Chapter 5), for example, naturally at considerable expense, instead of being told frankly to clean up your environment is in my opinion a very poor approach which does the patient little good in terms of long-term health. It isn't like visiting a regular doctor, where you merely take pills and forget about your complaint. You must *think* and work hard at eradication of those environmental factors which harm you. It is possible to build back good health, providing the bio-medical and physiological principles involved are properly understood and utilised. That is where I hope this book will help: to give you some understanding of what you are up against and how the various treatments work.

3

Have I Got Allergies?

You may be wondering if you have any allergies. The chances are you do. As you will see, minor degrees of intolerance are very common, though not serious. It depends whether you are ill or not. If you don't consider your health unduly impaired, the chances are that this phenomenon is unimportant to you, even if it could be demonstrated that it applies. But do remember the people surveyed by Dr Vicky Rippere and mentioned in chapter 1. They didn't regard themselves as ill but had several symptoms they considered normal. It is worth repeating the WHO definition of optimum health which is *complete physical, mental and spiritual well-being*. If your state of health doesn't meet this standard then you are, in a sense, ill. In actual fact that covers most of us. We live in a fascinating but complex world, our pace of life is hectic to say the least and we come into contact with large numbers of hostile substances which Nature never intended us to, so there is no doubt that the demands we place on our bodies are far too high. In fact it would be surprising if there were less illness than there is. The point about environmental disease is that although it is dramatically on the increase it can be counteracted, to a certain extent anyway. This is why it is worthwhile learning more about and why it repays the effort of studying it. There are many other causes of non-optimum health but allergies are amongst the easiest to put right.

Even if your complaints are trivial, the trouble is they may herald much more serious trouble later on. To ignore them now may be to do yourself a grave disservice. Unfortunately, there is no way of knowing in advance which cases will progress so, without making everyone paranoid about health (I use the term in its popular sense), I come again to the main theme of my book, which is that allergies concern us all.

With growing public awareness of the phenomenon of food and chemical intolerance more and more people have begun to wonder if they or members of their family might have allergies. How can you tell? This chapter should give you some guidance but it must be said that only a competent clinical ecologist can say with any certainty and only after an extensive interview and learning in considerable detail about diet and lifestyle before being able to make up his mind. Even then, he or she will tell you that final proof only comes from recovery due to avoidance of the offending substance or substances (see working definition of allergy in the previous chapter).

Nevertheless, there are a number of very helpful clues which bring about an immediate suspicion of maladaptation and these are worth considering in some detail. Always, the bulk of the diagnosis rests on the patient's account of himself (a very unpopular method of diagnosis in modern medicine, though it was heavily drummed into me and my colleagues at medical school that this was the 'correct' way to make one's diagnosis, at least initially).

Many symptoms and signs of allergic disease are to be found in ancient texts, so the condition has been around since time immemorial. Hippocrates himself refers many times to such phenomena and he seemed to be well aware of the importance of correct diet in health and disease. Indeed he writes sometimes of 'strong' and 'weak' foods and the capacity of the former to cause illness. The famous phrase 'One man's meat is another man's poison' goes back to Lucretius in ancient Rome and was originally intended in its literal, non-metaphorical, sense. So why has it taken so long for the idea to germinate in the minds of medical men? – it could hardly be said to have flowered, even now.

Well it is impossible to account for all the workings of the human mind but I submit that at least part of the reason is the men of science themselves enjoy eating enormously and are unwilling to consider the idea that it may be unhealthy for them. Probably they too are in the grip of food addictions. Indeed I have seen several of the outspoken critics of clinical ecology, and food allergies in particular, dramatising some of the effects given on the list below! Obviously it is hard to view objectively something which you yourself suffer from and the tendency is to regard many of these symptoms as 'normal' simply because one experiences them oneself.

TABLE OF SYMPTOMS

I make no apologies for reprinting here the table of allergy-based symptoms given in my first book (*The Food Allergy Plan*). It is a fascinating list in its own right and no book on ecology can stand alone without offering it as a superb insight into human illness. It should be written in letters of fire and taught to all medical students and prospective allied medical workers of every category.

It must be said immediately that many of the symptoms given below have other possible causes and are not proof positive of maladaptation disease. It is vital if you suffer from some form of illness and have not seen a doctor and had a proper diagnosis that you don't jump to conclusions. However if, as is usually the case, you have been ill for some time with no satisfactory explanation for the problem, despite tests and X-rays, and that the only treatment offered you has been the continued use of drugs to keep the symptoms at bay, then you are justified in assuming some or all of your symptoms may be due to maladaptation.

The more years you have had your symptoms, the less likely they are to signify a serious and progressive disease. The longer an illness continues, the more certain it is that it is not terminal! Yet some patients often worry unnecessarily, terrified lest they have cancer and the doctor is keeping this from them. Ironically, the doctor usually is holding something back; he doesn't know what is wrong and so can't give a satisfactory explanation, yet he is only human and seeks to cover up these deficiencies in his skills. This often has sinister overtones for the anxious patient.

The positive side of maladaptation disease is that, although unpleasant, it is reassuring. Firstly, you are not, as so many imagine, neurotic. Secondly, it is rarely life-threatening, except in certain special situations (asthma is one).

Symptoms may make life quite intolerable and many sufferers have seriously thought about committing suicide (I have no figures on how many actually do) but this is a special consideration. I am not being unsympathetic, merely stating what seems to be a fact: allergies don't kill. Life may be awful, but it goes on anyway.

In contrast to more chronic conditions, a disease which features relapses in short bursts and from which the patient tends to recover completely in between times, no matter how severe it may be when it strikes or how often it comes, is almost certain to be of an allergic nature. The fact that the victim is well between times means that there is little basically wrong with the individual or his body. It is adverse influences from without that result in repeated attacks.

However not all maladaptation syndromes follow this relapsing course. Remember if the offenders are frequently eaten, are even daily foods, there may be no opportunity to recover at all and the disease may seem to progress relentlessly, as in the case of arthritis for example.

This imposing list, by no means covering all possible subjective and bizarre symptoms of the kind described by Dr Ted

TABLE 3.1 SYMPTOMS ATTRIBUTABLE TO MALADAPTATION

The following symptoms are or may be attributable to maladaptation:

EYES	
red itchy eyes	blurring of vision
sandy feeling	spots in view
heavy eyes	flashing lights
dark rings	double vision (comes and goes)
unnatural 'sparkle'	'floaters'
watering	
EARS	
ringing in the ears	hearing loss
itching and redness of pinna	recurring infections, especially in children
earache	
CARDIO-VASCULAR	
rapid or irregular pulse	chest pain
palpitations, especially after eating	tight chest
blood pressure	pain on exercise (angina)
	feeling faint

TABLE 3.1 (*Continued*)

LUNGS	
tightness	hyperventilation (over-breathing)
wheezing	cough
poor respiratory function	
NOSE, THROAT AND MOUTH	
metallic taste	post-nasal drip
mouth ulcers	stuffed up
frequent sore throats	sinusitis
catarrh	stiffness of throat or tongue
sneezing	
GASTROINTESTINAL	
nausea	diarrhoea
dyspepsia	constipation
abdominal bloating	variability of bowel function
flatulence	hunger pangs
abdominal distress	acidity
pain in the stomach	
SKIN	
eczema	urticaria (hives)
rash that isn't eczema	excessive sweating
itching	chilblains
blotches	
MUSCULO-SKELETAL	
swollen painful joints	'rheumatism'
aching muscles	muscular spasms
stiffness	shaking (especially on waking)
cramps	pseudo-paralysis
fibrositis	
GENITO-URINARY SYSTEM	
menstrual difficulties	pressure
frequency of urination	genital itch
bedwetting	urgency
burning urination	
HEADACHE	
migraine	stabbing
sick headaches	solid feeling
pressure	mild or moderate headache
throbbing	stiff neck

TABLE 3.1 (*Continued*)

NERVOUS SYSTEM

inability to think clearly	memory loss
dopey feeling	stammering (attacks)
terrible thoughts on waking	maths and spelling errors
insomnia	blankness
crabby on waking	delusion
difficulty waking up	hallucination
bad dreams	desire to injure self
light-headedness	convulsions
twitching	

MENTAL STATE

STIMULATED, OVERACTIVITY

silliness	anxiety
intoxication	panic attacks
hyperactivity	irritability
tenseness	uncontrollable rage
restlessness	smashing-up attacks
fidgeting	general speeding up
restless legs	

DEPRESSED, UNDERACTIVITY

brain fag	depressed
withdrawn	lack of confidence
melancholy	unreal or depersonalised feeling
confused	low mood
crying	

HARD TO CLASSIFY BUT DEFINITELY REVEALING

sudden tiredness after eating	over- or underweight, history of fluctuating weight
sudden chills after eating	occasional swellings of face, hands, ankles, etc.
abrupt changes of state from well to unwell	persistent fatigue, not helped by rest
feeling totally drained and exhausted	vertigo
flu-like state that isn't flu	feeling unwell all over

(With acknowledgements to Theron Randolph, Richard Mackarness, Vicky Rippere and Marshall Mandell)

Hamlyn in Chapter 2, usually brings gasps of astonishment. Equally predictably, there are mutters and head-shaking signs of disapproval, scorn and disbelief from medical men when they are presented with it. Most of these 'symptoms' they claim are normal. Most people get them. True. But this doesn't mean they are correct and natural; common is not the same as normal or optimum. Also they are making a scientifically unsound assumption that most people don't have ay allergies. At best this is unproven but I hope by the time you finish reading this book you will have gained the conviction that an intelligent assessment of the facts leads inexorably to the conclusion that such an assumption is false.

VARIABILITY OF SYMPTOMS

In addition to the sheer diversity of symptoms is the baffling fact they they also come and go, moving from one part of the body to another, often in the same patient at different times, in any combination. Really, trying to find a pattern among groups of symptoms is hopeless. Dr Len McEwen has spotted one; he calls it PIMS, short for psychological disturbance, irritable bowel and migraine as a trio. It is one among many and it is doubtful that such groupings serve any purpose except to beguile others into thinking that more knowledge exists than is really the case. Fancy or technical sounding labels for diseases are one of the banes of modern medicine, akin to the abuses of 'Newspeak' from George Orwell's *Nineteen Eighty Four*, an attempt at propaganda by the redefinition of words.

It does a patient no good to be told that he has polymyalgia rheumatica or premenstrual tension. Such a label is a *symptom* and not an illness at all. Worse than that, it tends to deflect the physician from the fact that he hasn't a clue what he is dealing with. By assigning it a name there is the assumption that he has 'diagnosed' something – a patient might not care to hear that he is suffering from 'Mystery Disease No. 17' – and so the myth continues.

SHIFTING ILLNESS

Maladaptation disease also tends to vary over longer periods of time and this too has gone unnoticed by most medical observers.

Thus, for example, a child may have infantile eczema. The parents are told that he will 'grow out of it'. Sure enough, by about the age of seven years, the rash has gone. But then it turns into asthma. Later still this may have disappeared and the child now suffers from hay-fever or perhaps behavioural disorders. In adult life it may be migraine or arthritis. Yet all these disorders are really *one and the same complaint*: maladaptation to one or more common food or chemical.

Part of the difficulty lies in the fact that my colleagues are unable to recognise diseases such as arthritis and delinquency as allergic in origin, so of course they are not able to make these connections which are so helpful. But to those of us in the know it is easy to see, and so tragically frustrating that most doctors are unaware of this vital link in diagnosis which can lead to effective treatment.

TARGET OR SHOCK ORGANS

Why is it that the symptoms of allergy can be so diffuse and diverse? It is a question I am often asked. The answer lies in the concept of the target or shock organ. Allergic reactions, whatever their basis may finally be, are unquestionably disruptive to the body homeostasis (internal balance and orderliness). Our complex enzyme and biochemical systems, both extracellular and intracellular, require delicately balanced conditions, both physically and in terms of local concentrations of chemicals. Even a slight departure from these optimum conditions brings about a sharp deterioration in healthy operation. Thus, for example, quite tiny variations in pH, the body's acid/alkali status, are quite deleterious in consequences. In fact levels which would be of little significance in an inorganic system could be rapidly fatal to a living organism such as ourselves. Our bodies, fortunately, are provided with quite vigorous and effective correcting mechanisms to rectify departures from this optimum state and it is only when these mechanisms and the safety margins they bring are overwhelmed that symptoms ensue. Otherwise everything is put right without the problem ever coming to our attention (i.e. without symptoms).

It so happens that allergic reactions do sometimes produce enough disruption in this homeostasis, either generally or in specific parts of the body, to cause the safety mechanisms to fail.

This in turn diminishes the performance of any organ which is affected and the symptoms resulting are really a reflection of that malfunction, rather than the allergen causing it. Thus several different allergens can have the same effect in the same individual, if the same organ is affected. Conversely, the same allergen can have many different effects, if many organs in turn are disrupted.

Thus when the skin is affected, a rash may result. If the lungs feel the effect, an asthma attack will ensue. Bowel disturbance may lead to diarrhoea or colitis. Joint attack is recognised as painful movement and even 'arthritis'. And so on.

The part, or parts, of the body that seems to bear the brunt of the attack we call the target or shock organ and really the list of symptoms quoted above covers malfunction of just about every major organ of the body. Once this is understood, it is not very difficult to comprehend the disease process of a patient with multiple and mysteriously changing complaints. Doctors who don't know what they are dealing with however have tended to label these patients neurotic and consider such complex and Fabian illness to be psychosomatic. (The fact that they can't then explain what psychosomatic disease is either does not seem to deter many doctors from using this label!) This is a great tragedy. The doctor, naturally, is relieved of any burden and 'science' is satisfied, since there is now a diagnosis. But the sufferer is not served at all. It is an unkind and pompous label, assigning blame to the patient, instead of where it lies – with the physician who is ignorant of the matters described in this book and which were discovered many decades ago.

STRESS

This text is not meant to deny the existence of psychosomatic disorders. Undoubtedly these exist. But this is a diagnosis that must be made only *after* exhaustive search for possible environmental and nutritional causes for the disease process. At present this is rarely done, and there is ample evidence from a multiplicity of sources that there are very many people who, due to the omission of clinical ecology investigation procedures, are in mental hospitals and similar institutions when they need not be. Marshall Mandell, one of the world's leading research workers in this field, describes how he and William Phillpott, a likewise original thinker respected by clinical ecologists, spent several weeks treating a number of patients in a mental home, simply by attention to maladaptations.[1]

One of the problems which leads to confusion on this issue is the fact that stress does make symptoms worse in allergic patients. To the casual observer it may appear that stress causes the onset of symptoms, and so it does, in simple terms. But the stress is merely a trigger, the final straw in a sense, which takes effect only because of pre-existing allergic excitants which already have the body stretched to the point where there is no reserve in the homeostatic system. Typical of these cases, of which I have many, would be a person whose rash appears during bouts of marital tension. Once the ecologically safe diet is found and adhered to, the rash does not recur, despite the stress. In fact, in many such instances the marital tension may even resolve, as an added bonus, if it was due to chronic sickness in one of the partners!

Stress, whether it be a sudden acute illness, bereavement or a continuing personal conflict, influences allergic patients by lowering the individual's adaptation to his or her allergies. Thus, what may have been a Stage 2 *adapted* food suddenly becomes a Stage 3 maladapted one (see pages 42–3). Symptoms are inevitable unless this food is discontinued. Yet when the crisis has passed, that food may move back into being adapted and can then be tolerated once more. This shifting pattern frequently causes confusion. But it need not, once the basic principles are understood.

CEREBRAL ALLERGIES

The other great source of confusion which leads to the assumption that allergic manifestations may be psychosomatic is the fact that maladapted patients often behave in a strange manner, compute badly, have disturbances of mentation or hallucination and, in extreme cases, are completely out of reach mentally. Schizophrenia has been shown, on many occasions, to be allergic in origin, though it is doubtful if this covers all cases. Unfortunately, few doctors would see this disturbance of brain function as a clue to an ecological illness, especially in someone who was previously quite *compos mentis*.

In fact alterations in mentality are probably the commonest of all allergic manifestations. If you look again at the table of symptoms, you will see that those attributable to the nervous system or functional mentality form by far the largest group. Problems such as confused thinking, depersonalised feelings, low mood etc. are an almost invariable accompaniment to a maladaptation disease.

Minor degrees of these symptoms are quite common however and not confined to patients with allergies. People who consider themselves to be quite normal and healthy, experience such symptoms frequently or even daily. Irritability was experienced by 50 per cent of the subjects in Vicky Rippere's study of healthy normals, yet it is at times unquestionably an allergic response. Brain-fag, inability to concentrate and inexplicable low moods are so common as to be almost universal. To a clinical ecologist, this is ample demonstration that cerebral allergies are almost the rule, rather than the exception. This is not such a surprise when we consider that the brain is a very finely tuned organ and the communication point of our deepest psyche.

Common addictions which point to maladaptations and which are behind many instances of this brain dysfunction, are the social poisons such as tea, coffee and tobacco. Both tea and coffee contain caffeine and other methyl xanthine drugs. Yes drugs. These chemicals have a direct pharmacological action on the brain, kidneys and cardio-vascular system. Make no mistake, they are addictive. Like all poisons, they have first a stimulatory effect and then become depressors. In sufficiently large quantities, this depressor action becomes so severe as to cause cessation of function, in other words death. Very powerful toxins, such as cyanide, have an almost immediate lethal action. But strychnine, still very poisonous in small doses, in even smaller quantities acts as a stimulant and used to be included in many 'tonic' bottles.

Tea and coffee remain stimulants in the amounts that we are accustomed to. But drinking them is starting on the road to poisoning and for some people, especially those who like strong cups and indulge themselves frequently, there may be a very fine line between their daily intake and a real toxicity.

The addictive qualities of tea and coffee are easily observed in the usual beneficial effects to be derived from drinking them. Most people, if they are honest, will admit that if they go on too long without a 'fix' they begin to feel crabby and 'less than human'. These are but two examples among many. Wheat and milk seem to be almost equally addictive and are less often suspected. Few English meals, even snacks are without one or other of these foodstuffs and usually have both.

SOME DISEASES UNDER CONSIDERATION

As well as certain symptoms being highly suggestive of maladaptation illness, there are complete disease entities which suggest the possibility also. Asthma and eczema have long been known to be allergy-based disorders. But there are many others which, though not formally recognised as such, are frequently encountered (and remedied) by the clinical ecologists and are thus considered to be wholly or in part caused by allergies.

A provisional table is given below of such diseases. It is possible that as we learn more this list will be considerably extended in years to come.

Once again, it is important to stress that not all cases of these diseases may be helped by the clinical ecology approach. But a sufficient number of good recoveries are possible so that clinical ecologists feel it is mandatory to investigate such cases fully before embarking on costly, long-term drug therapy.

Some are more likely to be allergy-based than others. Thus, as we have seen from the Great Ormond Street study, migraine is more than 90 per cent likely to be due to food intolerance. If you add the possibility of non-dietary allergies that may mean

TABLE 3.2 DISEASE ENTITIES WHICH MAY HAVE SOME BASIS IN MALADAPTATION

Crohn's disease	anorexia nervosa
colitis	schizophrenia
migraine	depression
diabetes	hypertension
epilepsy	Menière's disease
arthritis, rheumatoid, osteo- and other	nephrotic syndrome
eczema	peptic ulcer
urticaria	alcoholism
neurasthenia	polymyalgia

that migraine is virtually a hundred per cent a maladaptation disease. On the other hand, epilepsy and nephrotic syndrome may only occasionally be helped to any marked degree by clinical ecology.

Alcoholism is not often recognised as a food allergy problem. But really tests indicate clearly that what the patient is addicted to is the ordinary food ingredient of his drinks – wheat, corn, yeast or sugar etc. It is simply that the alcohol causes it to be absorbed much faster and thus it is a more effective 'fix' for powerful cravings. Incidentally, hypoglycaemia, often inextricably bound up with food allergy, is another potent trigger for drinking. An alcoholic beverage provides a fast 'lift' for low blood sugar. Total elimination of offending foods will usually eradicate the cravings for drink, much to the relief of the addict. On the other hand, let an alcoholic with a maladaptation to wheat eat bread or a biscuit and he may suddenly find himself once again unable to resist the desire for beer or whisky. This cross-referencing of addictions makes the cure hopelessly fraught and difficult for alcoholics. Yet clinical ecologists can resolve it rather easily, though naturally we can do little about the underlying social stress which may have led to the addiction in the first place.

Hypertension might at first sight seem an unlikely runner, until you consider the fact that most people with high blood pressure are under stress and overweight. Obesity is caused by food addictions and addiction equals allergy, so there is a logical connection. All I can say is that in over 80 per cent of cases the blood pressure comes tumbling down on the Stone Age Diet (as given in the next chapter), without the use of drugs, which themselves create unpleasant side-effects (depression, impotence etc).

Diabetes may be another surprise but really it need not be. The common addictions in our society are to carbohydrate foods and we consume them to vast excess. Diabetes is known to be associated with this kind of dietary folly, probably because the pancreas gland becomes over-taxed and eventually exhausted. Remember also Professor Businco's work, quoted in chapter 1. It seems that any repeated stress, and allergic reactions are definitely stressful, ask a sufferer, can cause multiple non-specific damage to all organs. The pancreas, which has a host of complex functions to fulfil, hormonal and connected with digestion, is very vulnerable and, along with the adrenal gland, is one of the most consistently affected.

Believe it or not, it is illegal in this country to claim to be able to cure epilepsy. Happily, though, it is not against the law to tell you that convulsions are often demonstrably due to allergies. A fit is merely another symptom of temporary maladaptation. This is not surprising, bearing in mind what was written about cerebral allergies above. Most allergic reactions are either over- or under-functioning of an organ. A convulsion is really just a bout of extreme overactivity of the cerebral cortex and this is not essentially different from a skin rash, which is overactivity of the dermal cells, or diarrhoea, which is overactivity of the digestive system.

Several other of these diseases could be discussed along similar lines but lack of space precludes this. Instead you are referred to a number of more scholarly works given in the bibliography, if you are interested. Suffice it to say that the medical profession as a whole has a lot of revising of ideas to do. We do seem to be moving inexorably towards the assertion of Dr Albert Rowe that allergies are now the number one cause of illness in humans, now that microbial-based diseases are under control.

ADDICTION: A RIDE ON A ROLLER-COASTER?

One other aspect of the variability of symptoms in maladaptation which remains to be discussed is the cyclical pattern often observed. As you have read, allergic reactions are characterised by symptoms which depend on malfunction of various organs. These manifestations will differ in nature according to whether the organ in question is overstimulated or underperforming. An underfunctioning gut, for example, would be represented by constipation whereas, if overstimulated, diarrhoea might result.

It is possible to compile a table or ladder, showing the relative progression and recession of these symptoms. Dr Theron Randolph, doyen of clinical ecologists and premier in this aspect of maladaptation illness, has already done so[2] and his table is reproduced here with gratitude.

Two points need making clear. Firstly, there are no hard and fast gradations and these symptoms blend subtly one into another and indeed it is possible to have 'minus' reactions present at the same instant as 'plus' reactions. Secondly, each in-

TABLE 3.3 PRINCIPAL CLINICAL FEATURES OF VARIOUS STIMULATORY AND WITHDRAWAL LEVELS OF ALLERGIC DISTURBANCES

	Directions:	start at zero (0) Read up for predominantly Stimulatory Levels Read down for predominantly Withdrawal Levels
+ + + +	*Manic with or without convulsions*	Distraught, excited, agitated, enraged and panicky. Circuitous or one-track thought, muscle twitching and jerking of extremities, convulsive seizures, and altered consciousness may develop.
+ + +	*Hypomanic, toxic, anxious, and egocentric*	Aggressive, loquacious, clumsy (ataxic), anxious, fearful and apprehensive, alternating chills and flushing, ravenous hunger, excessive thirst. Giggling or pathological laughter may occur.
+ +	*Hyperactive, irritable, hungry and thirsty*	Tense, jittery, hopped up, talkative argumentative, sensitive, overly responsive, self-centered, hungry and thirsty, flushing, sweating and chilling may occur as well as insomnia, alcoholism, and obesity.
+	*Stimulated but relatively symptom free*	Active, alert, lively, responsive and enthusiastic with unimpaired ambition, energy, initiative and wit. Considerate of the views and actions of others. This usually comes to be regarded as 'normal' behavior.
0	*Behavior on an even keel as in homeostasis*	Children expect this from their parents and teachers. Parents expect this from their children. We all expect this from our associates.
–	*Localized allergic manifestations*	Running or stuffy nose, clearing throat, coughing, wheezing, asthma, itching, eczema and hives, gas, diarrhea, constipation colitis, urgency and frequency of urination, and various eye and ear syndromes.
– –	*Systemic allergic reactions*	Tired, dopey, somnolent, mildly depressed, edematous with painful syndromes (headache, neckache, backache, neuralgia, myalgia, myositis, arthralgia, arthritis, arteritis, chest pain), and cardiovascular effects.*
– – –	*Depressions and disturbed mentation*	Confused, indecisive, moody, sad, sullen, withdrawn or apathetic. Emotional instability and impaired attention, concentration, comprehension, and thought processes (aphasia, mental lapse, and blackouts).
– – – –	*Severe depression with or without altered consciousness*	Nonresponsive, lethargic, stuporous, disoriented, melancholic, incontinent, regressive thinking, paranoid orientation, delusions, hallucinations, sometimes amnesia, and finally comatose.

*Marked pulse changes on skipped beats may occur at any level.

dividual, though he or she may move around on the ladder tends to gravitate towards a permanent level which is appropriate to him or her. Even this 'chronic' level may move in time, usually ultimately tending towards the extreme minus end of the scale which represents total depletion of all body resources to oppose stress. So-called allergic reactions are thus, in reality, short-term departures from this chronic level.

Minus reactions are easy to equate with illness but the over-stimulatory phase is not, except in its extreme. Rather it is sometimes looked on as a good thing to be 'energetic', charging around all the time, 'getting things done'. Moreover, inappropriate laughter and enthusiasm tends to be viewed as evidence of a cheerful disposition when in fact it is merely a minor degree of intoxication, corresponding to a plus one or two reaction.

This table is a significant contribution to understanding your fellow men, illness apart, and it will amply repay careful study. You should be able to place your family and friends on it without much difficulty. Perhaps even yourself, if you can allow yourself to be objective enough. It is a great pity that it is not taught in medical schools, and all GPs and psychiatrists need to know it backwards, to avoid misdiagnosing and mistreating their patients.

The speed with which people can move from one phase to another is on occasion quite astonishing. I have seen patients, challenged with a food or chemical, appear excited, giggling and intoxicated yet within minutes be slumbering soundly, difficult to rouse. It is well known that for every 'high' there tends to be a corresponding 'low'. The transition can be sharp and the effect very unpleasant indeed. So much so that patients who have never touched alcohol can suffer alarming hangover symptoms. Indeed the inebriation effect caused by foods has remarkably been taken as drunkenness leading on occasion to unpleasant encounters with the police, who have taken a great deal of convincing, not surprisingly, when their own medical advisors have never heard of the problem.

YOUR SEX LIFE

Allergies may even have a part to play in your sexual activities. In much the same way that any body system can be stimulated and then depressed, so can sexual function. Reproduced below

TABLE 3.4 CHANGES IN SEXUALITY AT VARIOUS LEVELS OF REACTION

+ + + +	Performance commonly impossible
+ + +	Excessive desire: poorly co-ordinated performance
+ +	Hypersexuality in both desire and performance
+	Normal to slightly heightened sexuality
0	Normal
–	Normal to slightly reduced sexuality
– –	Debility and diminished desire and performance
– – –	Female frigidity and male impotence occur
– – – –	Frigidity and impotence the rule.

is another table, dealing with this aspect of physiology, again taken from the writings of Theron Randolph.[3]

Certain foods since time immemorial have been ascribed the power to increase sexual desire (aphrodisiacs). But as you see, any food may do it if the individual is maladapted to it and it produces a slightly enhanced reaction! Alcohol has always been the most potent of these foodstuffs, simply because by its nature it tends to provoke stimulatory reactions to the foods contained in the beverage. Those of you who know what brewer's droop is will understand that it also impairs function. Thus Shakespeare was right when he had the porter in Macbeth declare that alcohol 'provokes the desire, but it takes away the performance'. (Act 2 Scene 3).

It is interesting to speculate whether the present moral deterioration, known euphemistically as the permissive society, is not just a mass Stage Two Plus sexual reaction. Certainly it is timed coincident with a sharp decline in dietary standards which took place in the late fifties and early sixties, due to the vast increase in consumption of junk food and widespread addiction to carbohydrate sugary refined foods. It has also been shown that cats and other animals kept on bad diets often display homosexuality.

GLUE SNIFFING

One of the most distressing trends of addition to emerge recently is the habit of young people who seek kicks by sniffing potent organic solvents in the form of glues and aerosols. For a time, as with all poisons, there is a stimulatory phase and this brings them cerebral excitation and the kind of experience they desire.

The trouble is, with these extremely toxic substances, the margin between the 'effective' dose and outright poisoning is very small and danger is constantly present. This is in direct contrast to the remarks on tea and coffee earlier in this chapter.

Presumably the 'lucky' ones are those who find they move rapidly from the stimulatory to depressive phase. Rather than the sought-after thrill they are made nauseous and ill and soon abandon experimentation in favour of something else.

Youngsters who persist quite soon find themselves in a downward spiral of addiction, needing bigger and bigger doses to create any reaction and finally dangerous doses to have any effect at all. The end result is a Stage 3 maladaptation where bad symptoms are kept at bay only by further dosing of the substance. The usual fatality is someone who has progressed to this stage, rather than beginners. The practice of putting a polythene bag over the head and inhaling under it is especially dangerous and includes the risk of death by asphyxiation, as well as from poisoning.

Thixotropic glues seem to be very popular for this sort of activity. But other substances commonly in use include anti-perspirant sprays, butane gas canisters, lighter fluid and metal polish. (I came across the fact that metal polish as a sniffing substance has a history going back to the trenches in the First World War: soldiers who inhaled the polish supplied for their brassware found a certain 'lift', which presumably made it easier for them to face their appalling circumstances.)

The situation has become so alarming in the UK that it has now become illegal for retailers to sell these substances to young people, under penalty of heavy fines. It is a crude and rather unworkable attempt to deal with the problem, since the cause of this latest craze is not the retailer. Therefore the wrong target has been selected.

Treatment for the individual rests not only with getting him or her to kick the habit, which will be very difficult in the absence of any other help, but a full ecological 'clean up' of the environment, at school and at home (see Chapter 10). Diet will need to be examined for allergens and these removed. In addition common chemicals around the house would need to be replaced with safer substances, not to prevent temptation, but to avoid constant provocation of Stage 3 maladaptation/withdrawal symptoms by substances which are chemically similar.

4

Tracking Down Hidden Food Allergies

While on a trip to Japan recently, a friend of mine, Dr Yukio Kitajima of the Kohsei Chuo hospital in Tokyo, surprised me by introducing me to the 'Chinese Method' of diet therapy. As he explained it to me it was basically a mixture of elimination and rotation dieting, as covered below, and showed a clear-cut understanding of the manifestations of food allergies, though apparently without using such a term. It is very old and goes back many centuries.

Here in the West one of the earliest references to an allergy-effective diet, though again without actually calling it such, is in a treatise by the Italian nobleman Luigi Cornaro, written in 1550, 'A Sober and Temperate Life'. He discourses on diet and emphasizes eating moderately. It was always his practice to rise from the table slightly unsatisfied. Remember, this was in an age when gluttony, especially among the aristocracy, was the norm.

But more interestingly still, he set out to discover the foods which suited him best and then stuck to those. In other words, he worked out and kept to his own elimination diet. He questioned the assumption that what is good for the palate must be good for the stomach and he reports: 'The issue was that I found it to be false: for though rough and very cold wines, as likewise melons and other fruits, salad, fish and pork, tarts, garden-stuff, pastry and the like, were very pleasing to my palate, they disagreed with me notwithstanding'.[1]

Before embarking on his plan, Cornaro ate and drank liberally, as did his peers but he finally experienced a complete breakdown of health and spirits by the time he was forty and was, indeed, lucky to survive. Yet he was able to rescue himself simply by changing his dietary and other habits. The success of his elimination plan was such that he cured himself of his severe illness and went on ultimately to live to the grand age of 99.

FOOD ALLERGIES COME FIRST

Following the theme of this book, that food allergies are widespread and that most people, if not all, have one or two at least, this could be said to be a most important chapter. True, if the person isn't ill in the strict sense of the word, it may not seem worthwhile going through some of the procedures, which could be more demanding than his or her state of health warrants. But the Stone-Age Diet is easy to follow, once having got used to it, and it may reveal startling improvements in what was supposed to be normal health. Certainly if the individual finds it tough going to follow a restrictive diet, that itself is evidence of food addictions, i.e. allergies. Perhaps everyone should give it a try at some time or other during their lives. Certainly beyond, say, 35 when stress will have taken some toll of the body's optimum functions and intolerances may come to the fore. Often an increasingly poor performance is attributed to advancing years yet, as Luigi Cornaro demonstrated, advancing age *of itself* does not automatically lead to dulling of the mind and body. You might be pleasantly surprised!

Food allergies remain the most important aspect of maladaptation disease, largely because we eat much larger quantities of food than we inhale of chemicals or dusts etc. From the therapeutic point of view also, they assume maximum importance because it is relatively easy to detect and correct food allergies, compared to the situation with inhalant allergens such as dust or atmospheric chemical pollution. The question of total body burden enters here: often we are able to cope with a certain amount of intolerance to food and chemicals, it is only when this overall tolerance is exceeded that symptoms begin to occur. Thus if we tackle the relatively easy job of finding and removing food allergens, this may mean that the body is able to recover sufficiently so that further explorations are not necessary.

If you are going it alone, more exact details of these procedures are given in my book *The Food Allergy Plan*. You might care to show your doctor a copy of that book, or the present one, and seek his or her co-operation, if not actual interest.

It should be said that no practising clinical ecologist will succeed for long without adopting broadly the methods given here. Thus even if you go to the expert, you will probably encounter these or similar techniques and it will help you to understand what is going on. Subsequent chapters cover other methods of identifying and treating allergies, but dietary manipulations remain paramount at all times.

SINGLE FOOD ELIMINATIONS

This is the least satisfactory method of identifying food allergies and is most unlikely to succeed, except by sheer luck. Dr Doris Rapp (USA) calls in the analogy of eight nails sticking up in a shoe: if only one of the nails is removed, the victim will still limp. It is rather like that with allergies. You must remove all – or certainly most – at once, in order to notice any improvement.

You may be quite certain that you are allergic to coffee and avoid it strictly, only to find it makes no difference. The fatal error is then to assume you cannot be allergic to that food and go back to eating or drinking it! You may have been right in the first place but there were simply a number of other allergies present at the same time.

This does not detract from the fact that omitting a specific food does sometimes produce miraculous recoveries. It is simply that it is such a hit and miss method it has nothing to commend it in systematically tracking down food allergy as a cause of ill-health.

FASTING

Fasting as a health technique has a long and often quasi-religious tradition. However Theron Randolph, of Chicago, refined it as a clinical ecology method, based on his understanding of the mechanisms of masked allergies. He is without equal as a teacher in this field and we all owe a great deal of our present knowledge to him and his persistence, in the face of the most vitriolic and uninformed criticism from his colleagues, in studying the phenomena of maladaptation and experimenting with different methods of treatment. His experience now spans many decades.

There is a certain satisfying logic to fasting. If the patient feels well it is definitely a food allergy; conversely, if not, the diagnosis becomes unlikely. Patients often feel wonderful on a fast and many of them say glumly, 'If only I didn't need to eat!'

All food is avoided for a period of four days minimum, only spring-water being taken. Smoking is forbidden, naturally (tobacco is one of the commonest of all hidden allergies). Less than four days is virtually useless, since all foods must void from the bowel before any firm conclusions can be drawn, though in fact some people feel well in less time than this.

Usually, however, the first two or three days are a time of exacerbation of symptoms. Just as an alcoholic feels ill when he stops drinking, so too can the fasting patient experience very unpleasant effects by cutting off food suddenly. Remember from Chapter 2 that allergy and addiction are often identical. These are called withdrawal symptoms. Fasts of one or two days often result in feeling bad *because they don't go on long enough*. The withdrawal symptoms never have time to clear. Contrary to expectations, after several extra days, the patient feels a sparkling return to health, a resurgence of energy and loss of fatigue. Since this depends on the bowel clearing itself of all food residues, taking Epsom salts or some other laxative may assist in this process.

If after five to seven days the patient is no better, then food allergy is not the cause of illness. The only rare exception is someone who also reacts strongly to chemicals and other environmental factors, which keep him ill, even though he has some food intolerance. It is advisable therefore to fast in controlled surroundings, avoiding such extraneous factors as plastics, traffic fumes, perfumes, dusts, pets etc.

The point about a fast is that it not only may point the way to a cure. It will also *unmask* hidden food allergies. That means that after the five days have elapsed and if symptoms have cleared the opportunity presents itself to test each food singly, with the expectation that each allergenic food will provoke a response of some kind. The masking effect will not come into play and disguise the reaction.

Thus foods are returned to the diet *one at a time*, starting on the morning of the fifth day. Two or three foods a day may be introduced. Those which are safe may be retained in the diet, those which are not are discarded. The pulse is counted before and after each test feed. Those which increase the pulse or cause irregularities are highly suspect.

The problem is, if symptoms are provoked the patient must then wait until they have subsided before trying the next test. Although disappearance of these symptoms may be speeded by taking bicarb and Epsom salts (see above), it may take one or two days at worst. So the first foods tested must be those most unlikely to produce a reaction. In that way a number of foods can be added to the diet and retained as safe. Salmon, rabbit, mangoes and other uncommon foods are usually suggested for the first two days.

Later, more suspect foods are used. If one reacts, no new food may be tried until symptoms have gone *but those already proven safe are retained*. Last of all come the problematical foods, such as milk, wheat, sugar, coffee etc., which are highly likely to cause trouble.

Some clinics rely heavily on fasting. In my own practice we rarely use it, except for specific situations where it is indicated and these are not common. The reason is that it needs close supervision. Taking the patient into a special ward would be ideal. A further difficulty which makes me cautious is that after avoiding all foods it then may be difficult for the patient to find anything to eat which does not cause a reaction. I have sometimes had patients trapped in this way, usually the multi-allergics and these are precisely the cases where one is sometimes tempted to suggest a fast. It does appear that unmasking all food simultaneously is risky and a significant objection to this method. Perhaps admission to a controlled ecological environment (see Chapter 6) is the answer; chemical exposures can be regulated at the same time.

For certain patients fasting is definitely ill-advised for self-help and diagnosis. Subjects for whom it is especially unsuitable are:

1. diabetics on insulin;
2. asthmatics;
3. very debilitated cases;
4. those who have had an anaphylactic reaction;
5. epileptics;

6. those suffering from extreme emotional disturbance or who have ever contemplated suicide.

It is important to understand that the effects of challenging a newly unmasked allergy can be quite extreme. Patients are often astonished how bad these reactions may be. Medical help should always be readily available.

THE HALF FAST

The half fast is a term I made up myself. It seems to describe admirably extreme diets, such as lamb and pears, which are really a compromise with fasting. The Cambridge group, studying irritable bowel syndrome, referred to in Chapter 2, allowed the patient to choose one meat, one fruit and one vegetable. Fish and rice may be used.[2] A grape diet, eating only grapes, is similar. There are numerous others.

All are subject to the same risk – if one of the allowed foods happens to be an allergen the whole (considerable) effort is wasted. The patient will not get well. True, with so few foods the chances of one of them being an allergen is small. Especially since relatively safe foods are chosen.

The reason for the compromise is simple – to be kind to the patient and to avoid the need for complete avoidance of food, which is tougher psychologically than it is physically. But it seems to me that it incorporates the risk of failure, such as may be present using broader diets, with the great demands made of the patient that a fast engenders; a marriage of two difficulties.

About the only situation where it is regularly preferred by me is in cases of colitis and Crohn's disease (regional ileitis), where in truth the trouble is just as likely to be fruit, meat and vegetables as it is wheat, coffee and all the usual difficult foods. Even then, I like to improve the chances of success by testing for safe combinations of foods, using the provocation-neutralisation method, as described in Chapter 5.

THE STONE-AGE DIET

Health food fans are constantly in search of Man's optimum or most natural diet. The Hunzas of the Himalayas are supposed to exemplify good eating: certainly they are famous for their longevity. Vegetarians think their way is best and 'healthiest'. Vegans are more extreme but just as assured. There are many groups and many different points of view on what we should eat to be 'correct'.

Richard Mackarness, former consultant psychiatrist at Basingstoke Hospital and now world-famous clinical ecologist, thinks archaeology provides the answer. He went in search of what our ancestors used to eat, as evidenced by dentition, faecal waste and kitchen middens unearthed by archaeologists from prehistoric periods. He came up with what he called the Stone-Age Diet, or sometimes the Caveman Diet, which he started to use to treat certain mentally ill people.[3] Certainly it seems logical. In essence his diet consists of meat, fish, fruit and vegetables, water to drink. If you think about it, that's just about what our primitive nomadic ancestors would have eaten; it is a hunter–gatherer diet.

Only since we (the human race) settled and became farmers did we introduce foods such as wheat and cereals, eggs on a regular basis and dairy produce. This has only been in the last ten thousand years or so. In other words they are not strictly speaking *natural* foods. And what do you know – these are very *common allergy* foods! It seems that we are not well adapted to them as yet.

Along came alcohol; then, a few centuries ago, we added sugar and stimulant drinks; more recently refined carbohydrate and finally, in the last few decades, food chemical additives and crop-sprays, and of course these are not natural either. All these substances feature prominently amongst food allergies.

Whether or not the hypothesis is correct – that this is what our ancestors ate – it works remarkably well as a hypo-allergenic diet.

If you wish to try the Stone-Age Diet for yourself, it is outlined in the table below. Follow it for about two weeks before making up your mind as to whether or not it has any benefit for you. If you feel partly or wholly better it is good presumptive evidence of allergies to one or more of the banned foods.

If you feel better on the diet it only remains to identify which foods had been making you ill. To do this, you must reintroduce each food substance *one at a time*. Those which seem to have no

THE STONE-AGE DIET

You may not eat

Dairy produce, including butter, most margarines, cheese, cream yoghurt, skimmed milk and even goat's milk;

Cereals, including wheat, barley, corn, rice, oats and rye, nor any flours or derivatives of these (such as bread, cakes, biscuits, pastry etc.);

egg or chicken (turkey, duck and other fowl are allowed);

sugar, honey or sweeteners;

tea, coffee, alcohol or tobacco;

citrus fruits;

cures, remedies, pills and potions except life-saving drugs such as insulin, digoxin and thyroid hormone;

tap water;

manufactured foods of any kind, from packets, tins, jars, bottles etc. All these usually contain additives (chemicals) and adulterants (such as wheat, sugar and corn). Definitely out. Think twice even about vinegar, mustard etc.

You may eat

fresh meat;

fresh fish;

fresh fruit;

fresh vegetables;

spring or bottled water;

herb teas;

nuts;

certain fruit juices, namely apple, grape and pineapple, those without any additives of any kind;

frying is allowed, including chips, but use only sunflower or safflower oil.

effect may be retained. Those which provoke a reaction should be omitted, of course.

This is explained in more detail in the following section.

INDIVIDUAL FOOD CHALLENGE TESTS

Eating a portion of food to see if it causes a reaction is called challenge feeding. It is vital to unmask a food allergy before attempting to do this test, otherwise the results are meaningless. As Randolph, Rinkel and Zeller state:

> Actually, the most discerning patient is rarely ever able to detect the

presence of a masked food allergy. In fact the most skilled allergist cannot do so either until he tests for it. Masking may be 100% perfect, even with an individual food test, if steps have not been taken to avoid it.[4]

If you wish to test a food you are at present eating, do not eat it for at least four days, preferably five, before testing. Naturally, if you have been on the Stone-Age Diet for a longer period, all banned foods qualify for this test.

The correct procedure for these challenge tests is given in *The Food Allergy Plan* but can be summarised briefly here:

1. Test only on a day when you are feeling well. If, for example, you are still undergoing a reaction to a food tested the day before, wait until it clears up before proceeding.
2. Eat only the food you are interested in for the test meal. Spring water and salt (if needed) are permitted. Nothing else. Eat a substantial portion, to be sure of provoking any reaction.
3. Eat the food raw or prepared only very simply. Compound foods (mixtures) are not allowed. Only single food items. It is best to procure these free of any chemical contamination, if possible. If not, carry out the test anyway.
4. Lunchtime is the best meal. If you use the evening meal it is possible to sleep through an allergic reaction and miss it. This way, if symptoms occur in the afternoon, you can be fairly certain the food was to blame. Conversely, if there are no symptoms at all, you then eat a normal evening meal but include more of the test food. If no symptoms are experienced by next morning, you are justified in treating it as a safe food.
5. It is possible to increase the accuracy of this procedure by including a pulse count. Arthur Coca, in his controversial little book *The Pulse Test*,[5], reported the fact that allergic contacts may on favourable occasions increase the pulse rate markedly. The heart-rate may also become very irregular and this too is diagnostic of an allergic reaction following on a challenge feed. His method gained little general acceptance but he considered it provided sufficient worthwhile information to be quite helpful. What he didn't realise was that unmasking – which wasn't then a recognised phenomenon – increases the likelihood of a pulse reaction and so, in effect, adds measurably to the success of his technique.

A resting pulse is taken before and after the test meal, actually two or three times afterwards, say thirty and sixty minutes later. By resting pulse is meant that the patient sits still for two minutes before counting. A rise or fall of ten or more beats after challenging is considered highly suggestive of an allergy and it is best to avoid such foods, even in the absence of overt symptoms on test.

It is sensible when testing a Food for the first time to *smell and taste* it before committing yourself. Animals do this all the time: you may notice a dog sniffing and licking any unknown substance before ingesting it. They follow their instincts as to whether or not a substance is safe to eat. Nature knows best! Humans can also easily learn to develop this faculty. If when you smell it or taste a little you get a distinct negative impression, *don't* make yourself ill by eating the whole portion!

THE BUILD UP EFFECT

Occasionally, with certain patients, it takes more than one or two challenge doses to bring on a reaction, even if the food is inimical to that individual. Patients talk of a 'build up'. It seems that infrequent or well-spaced doses can be tolerated to a degree (indeed, this is the basis of the rotation diets given below). Thus testing can fail and unnoticed allergens pass back into the diet, to wreak havoc.

The way to overcome this obstacle, if it is suspected, is both simple and obvious: have the patient eat the food continuously for several days, before assessing its effect. If symptoms come on after forty-eight hours, or so, then that food must be an allergen, providing all other variable factors (such as environmental chemicals) are kept constant during that time.

The main problem with doing it this way is that the patient may be finding dietary restrictions very irksome and he or she may be desperate to get back onto a more 'normal' diet. It is going to take far longer reintroducing one or two foods per week than it would at the rate of only one a day. Of course I always point out that the very foods desired so urgently are probably harmful and craved because of addictions.

On the plus side, foods found to be bothersome only with cumulative eating need not necessarily be strictly avoided but can be rotated every four or five days. Patients who have this sort of result in testing are probably ideal for the rotation diet method given below.

CYCLICAL AND FIXED ALLERGIES

Patients are occasionally baffled by the behaviour of allergies when testing. For example, a food may be tested and found entirely satisfactory and yet within two weeks that same food clearly emerges as a source of new problems. Alternatively, a food may have dire consequences on occasion, yet some time later appear to be relatively harmless.

The key to this shifting pattern and an important principle to grasp in connection with testing foods is that of cyclical and fixed allergies, first discovered by Herbert Rinkel in the 1930s. Consequently these are explained here. However it is important to understand that this mechanism applies not only to foods but to chemicals and inhalant allergens also.

Fixed allergies, as the name implies, never really change. Once acquired they last for life. In general fixed allergies are severe. These are probably immunologically induced and, in accordance with our present understanding at any rate, there is no reason to expect them to alter. If antibodies are involved, as in the IgE mediated or immediate hypersensitivity (Type 1) response, these will always be available in the future to react with the allergen (antigen). However, not all fixed allergies are of the immune-based type.

Cyclical allergies, on the other hand, vary considerably in their propensity to induce reactions. The more frequent the encounter, the more pronounced the reactions which result. In terms of a food, this means the more often it is eaten, the greater power of devastation it acquires. If it is avoided for a period, the allergenicity diminishes and so do the resultant symptoms.

The actual period of avoidance varies a great deal. In some cases as little as a few days may result in loss of response to a single mild dose. Others may require many months of strict avoidance. The majority lie somewhere in between. If, after two years, a response is still detectable, Theron Randolph considers it justifiable to shift that particular allergen into the category *fixed*.

This is highly relevant to challenge testing. The optimum interval between avoidanceand testing is five to ten days. Five days are needed for unmasking but, beyond that time, the sooner the tests are carried out, the better. After ten days, certain allergens may begin to lose their effect and so be missed on the single challenge feed. As a result the patient may consider it a safe food, eat it frequently and suffer a baffling exacerbation of symptoms.

This cycling nature of certain allergens has its advantageous side also. What is at one moment a food that must be avoided at all costs months later may easily be tolerated, at least in small and infrequent doses. This is obviously preferable to life-long avoidance. Thus resting of foods (or any allergen) has important benefits. Conversely, frequent and especially daily consumption of any one food item is considered inadvisable. It could lead to the development of new allergies. Though not universal, this is a major problem for some patients and must be guarded against if they are to maintain health. That leads on naturally to the next section, which is how to avoid developing new allergies.

ROTATORY DIVERSIFIED DIETS

Hardly surprisingly, the principle of rotating foods was first propounded by Herbert Rinkel, who discovered the cyclical nature of most allergies. The rules for devising your own rotation diet are really quite simple:

1. Eat only fresh whole foods. Most manufactured food is adulterated, that is containing foreign ingredients. There is little use in avoiding or rotating a food like wheat if you eat a beefburger which contains it in a hidden form. Corn is probably the most widespread agent used in this fashion and can usually be recognised on the packaging label as modified food starch etc. But there are many others.

So far as is possible, avoid those substances which are chemically contaminated. Unfortunately, this is hardly possible with modern commercial supplies. Even vegetables and fruit are covered with insecticides, weed-killer and fertilisers. To obtain organic supplies is not impossible but certainly difficult. Perhaps the best advice is to do what you can. Only extreme cases need to go to extreme lengths.

Published lists of organic growers and suppliers exist. Action Against Allergy, 43 The Downs, London SW20 8HG or similar action groups should be able to help by providing names and addresses.

2. Vary your diet. Diversity is the key to success. Eating the

same few foods over and over again is one of the reasons allergics get into difficulties in the first place. In our Western diet, most dishes contain wheat, milk, sugar or egg; often several or all of them. Basically it is a highly monotonous diet but due to the fact that the ingredients are well-disguised and inventively cooked this point is often overlooked.

It is necessary for allergics to take in many more foods than most of us. It occurs to me that one of the reasons we are developing more allergies than formerly is this very monotony of eating. Owing to our storage and preparation methods, the same foods are available more or less the year round. Formerly, when we were much more tied to local farming, people ate largely what was available and that would vary according to season. Thus at certain periods there would be a glut of cabbages, lettuce, roots, fruit and so on. Doubtless these foods were overeaten at times of excess; but then a new crop would come in and that in turn would take over predominance in the diet. Few foods, except grains, could be stored the whole year round and consequently Nature herself would impose a kind of rotation which, while not as strict as the sort given here would certainly help to prevent intolerance developing, or terminate the effects if it did.

Those who live in cities have it far easier of course. There are many cosmopolitan communities now existing within the city boundaries. Each of these tends to import ethnic foods that suit them and, collectively, this offers a tremendous diversity of choice, even if prices come a little higher than indigenous foods. Chinese, Pakistani and Middle Eastern shops are particularly good in this respect. Delicatessens may help also.

3. Rotate foods. The minimum useful period for rotation is four days. Less than that and the food just does not have time to clear the bowel before the next dose and masking could result.

Five days is only slightly harder to fill. A week has the attraction that each calendar day has the same menu, which makes it easy to remember. But more safe foods are required and the patient may not have a sufficient number of these.

An example of a four-day rotation diet is given below. It is merely a suggestion and need not be slavishly copied. Omit any foods which you know for certain cause symptoms and substitute others of your preference (having regard to food families, as described in *The Food Allergy Plan*). Listed foods

TABLE 4.1 FOUR-DAY ROTATION DIET

Food	*Day 1*	*Day 2*	*Day 3*	*Day 4*
Meat	lamb	pork	beef	chicken
Fish	plaice sole etc	cod haddock etc.	trout salmon	mackerel tuna
Veg	cauli beans	carrots celery	cabbage peas	parsnip onion tomato lettuce
Fruit	apple pears	grape	banana stone fruit	melon pineapple
Drink	apple juice	grape juice	tea	pineapple juice
Filler	Ryvita	oatcakes	bread	potato
Misc.	peanuts soya milk	sultanas raisins brazil nuts	milk walnuts and pecans	egg hazelnuts or cashews

may be repeated at least once during the permitted day. It should work well for moderately allergic individuals.

A seven-day diet operates on the principle one food – one meal – one day in seven. In other words each food is only ever eaten once in seven days and not in conjunction with any other food. This is harder to do and such diets are highly personalised, depending on individual sensitivities. It needs twenty-one foods and is really only for severe cases who react to just about everything, so-called universal reactors (Total Allergy Syndrome, so beloved of the media).

The question remains: are such diets nutritionally adequate? Certainly they are borderline. But it is encouraging to know that in a test on laboratory fed rats, those given short rations on average lived half as long again as those given generous food supplies. Your attention is also drawn once again to the 'temperance' principle of Cornaro at the start of this chapter.

Clearly there is more to nutrition than what Ross Hulme Hall calls 'adding machine' dietetics.

Theron Randolph thinks such diets are balanced.

> There is an adequate amount of carbohydrate, calories, protein, and other food constituents over the course of a week to maintain health. Does the patient get enough vitamins and minerals on such a diet? In my experience, the consumption of whole (and especially organic) foods, served fresh, will provide better nutrition than the average American diet, even when the latter is supplemented by vitamin pills. In general, I do not recommend vitamin supplements to patients on this diet . . . I am not against vitamins – far from it. But I believe it is always preferable to obtain vitamins from their natural source, in whole foods, rather than through a supplement, which may contain traces of various chemicals or foods, including additives (corn starch, milk lactose and so forth) that can aggravate allergic problems.[6]

It may not be my place to disagree with my mentor but I do regard it as difficult, if not impossible, to get adequate vitamin and mineral supplies from food that is currently available. Often forced farming methods and soil that is exhausted result in crops which are deficient in basic ingredients, such as used to be present in our food. A number of companies now, aware of the problem, are seeking to produce hypo-allergic vitamin and mineral supplements, free of corn, sugar, colourings and other noxious ingredients.

The bottom line is that an allergic patient may react to any and every product, for one reason or another and in that Randolph is right.

SPECIALISED DIETS

There are a number of well-known diets intended to meet particular needs. For example Dr Dong's diet for arthritis sufferers has helped many cases to ease or eradicate their problems. Basically, the diet may be summarised as avoiding the following foods:

red meat
fruit, including tomatoes
dairy produce
egg yolks
vinegar or any other acid

pepper
chocolate
alcohol
any manufactured food with additives, preservatives, colourings etc. of any kind.

It is notable that this diet allows wheat, tea and coffee, a liberty which any clinical ecologist would view askance (very common allergens, see tables below).

Campbell has another version, which allows milk but bans wheat. (I would take care to ban *both*!)

The trouble with all such diets is three-fold. To begin with no one diet could possibly help every case and often this isn't made clear. Secondly, apparently unaware of the behaviour of food allergens, most authors omit to make the point that the diet may help temporarily and then begin to fail, due to developing *new* allergies. Rotating foods would cure this. Finally, the patient is not told how to work out which foods are the culprits, as explained under food challenge tests above. It is wrong of course to assume that all foods banned are equally guilty, even if the diet does succeed.

ENZYME SUPPLEMENTS

At least one theory of food allergy is that digestion of food is inadequate, which leads to characteristic proteins being absorbed into the blood. These are foreign proteins and stimulate the immune system to react.

If the food were properly broken down to its constituent parts (simple sugars, fatty acids and amino acids of low molecular weights) then, so the theory goes, these would not be large enough molecules to trigger the immune system and so allergic reactions would not take place.

In practice it does seem to be helpful to give food allergics supplements of digestive enzymes. Dr. William Philpott pioneered this method in the USA. The stomach pH (acidity) needs to be correct and this can be tested with indicator paper touched to the saliva. Hydrochloric acid tablets are used, if required, or bicarbonate of soda. A mixture of animal-extracted pancreatic enzymes follows and this contains most of the powerful digestive enzymes which work on food.

Thus even if the individual is deficient in production of own secretions, the breakdown process can take place efficiently with assistance.

It is only partially successful, and not in all cases, so the theory must only be part of the story. Nevertheless, it is an attractive idea and fits in with our understanding of physiology.

For some patients it means the difference between success and failure.

FREQUENCY OF FOOD ALLERGIES

It might be of interest, before closing this chapter on the management of food allergies by direct manipulation of diet, to provide a table of frequencies of different food allergies. A number of studies have been done over the years and slightly varying results may be obtained, depending on the group studied, the country and the exact questions asked. However the general picture seems to be remarkably consistent.

Professor Soothill's group, studying migraine children at the Great Ormond Street Hospital, gave the following distribution for food allergies (remember 93 per cent of these children were found to be intolerant to one or more foods and that this was the basis of their migraines):

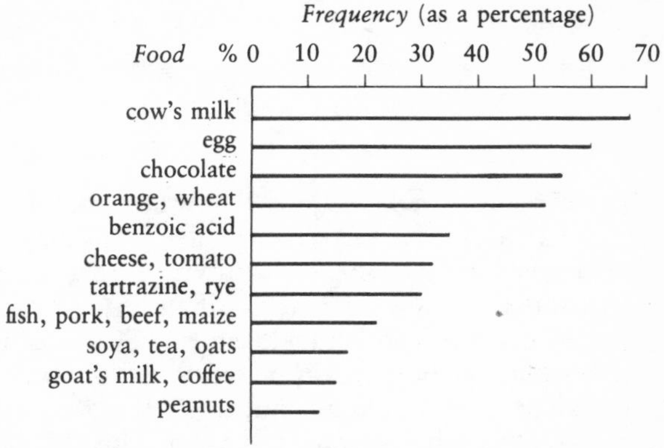

Fig. 4 *Frequency of Causative Agents (Foods) of Migraine in Children*

Dr Vicky Rippere, a clinical psychologist at the London Institute of Psychiatry, carried out a survey of eighty-five people with known food and chemical intolerances. Over 95 per cent were allergic to foods and she uncovered the following distribution of frequencies (adult patients, twenty males and sixty-five females):

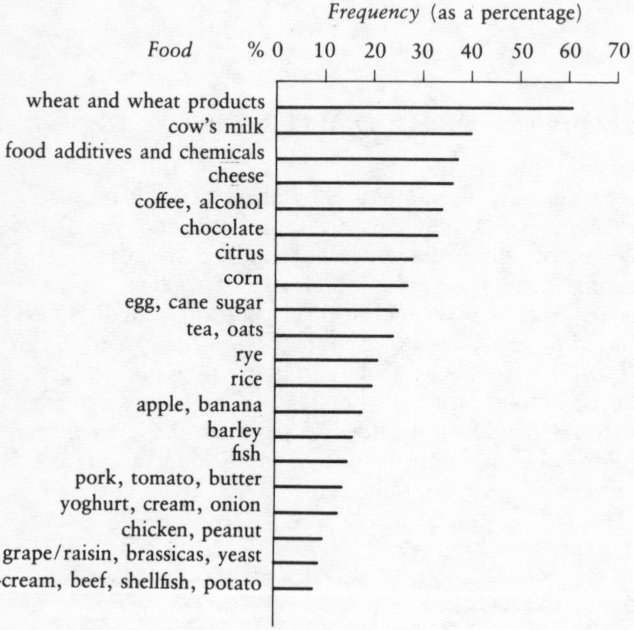

Fig. 5 *Frequency of Food Allergies in a Group of Adult Patients*

This might be considered the adult 'top twenty'. Monosodium glutamate, soya and beet sugar are just outside this table. Probably all practising clinical ecologists would agree that yeast is far too low. It probably belongs in the first half-dozen or so. The reason it is not reported with such frequency is probably that it rarely occurs alone but usually in combination with other offenders, such as bread or in alcohol.

Note that children differ slightly at the top. This is fairly consistent with other workers' findings. Corn is a very prominent allergy among children, largely because it is used as a sugar in soft drinks, squashes and sweets and is also consistently added to what is usually called 'junk' food as a starch bulker.

5

Skin Testing For Allergies

The first allergy skin test on record goes back to the case of Lady Hannage in 1603. She was lady-in-waiting to Queen Elizabeth I and asked to be excused certain of her duties due to an allergy to roses. Evidently she was mistrusted because someone laid a rose petal on her cheek while she was asleep. Perhaps fortunately for her, a blister duly appeared and she proved her case.

In 1656 Pierre Borel, who was also one of the pioneer microscopists, confirmed a patient's hypersensitivity to egg by applying some to the skin and observing the resultant blister.

Classic experiments were carried out in 1873 by Charles Blackley of Manchester. He demonstrated that pollen allergy lay behind hay-fever by inhalant tests which produced the typical catarrhal symptoms, and by rubbing pollen on a scratch in the skin, which resulted in large urticarial wheals. He carried out the tests on himself. In order to make his case more complete he collected pollens on gelatine plates exposed to the breeze and showed that large collections on the plates coincided with the times of maximum symptoms in sufferers (the basis of today's 'pollen count'). He even mounted his plates on kites and sent them up to 500 metres high but still found plenty of pollen. Unfortunately, he was years ahead of his time. Like many other great observations and experiments, his work was completely ignored for decades.[1]

SKIN PRICK OR SCRATCH TESTS

Modern prick or scratch tests, using the skin for identifying allergens, began with doctors Noon and Freeman in 1911. Typically, these are used to demonstrate a Type I hypersensitivity reaction which gives a wheal and flare response. Type III is characterised by an oedematous swelling though not invariably. Type IV reactions are usually much delayed and may be read next day, as opposed to immediately.

Generally, these latter slower reactions are best identified by patch testing. A pad of material soaked in the antigen is held in continuous contact with the skin for a period of twenty-four hours or more. There must be a control test carried out simultaneously, to exclude false positive results. If the site of the patch containing the solution shows significant reddening and swelling, as opposed to the control which has none of the active ingredient, the test is considered positive.

Conventional intradermal skin tests are carried out using extracts of materials which may be inhaled or eaten, such as dust danders, pollen and food. The tests are carried out by placing a drop of solution on the skin and then scratching or pricking the skin under this. Alternatively, the test may be performed by injecting a small quantity of the antigen intradermally, though the latter is considered less safe. The solutions are usually quite dilute, 1:20 strength or less. Several are introduced to the skin at the same time, up to two dozen being not uncommon.

A control test using neutral fluid is performed at the same time. It is customary to mark the skin with boxes and label tags, such as letters or numbers, to keep track of which site is which antigen.

A positive result is read with reference to the control result. If, after fifteen to twenty minutes, the suspect allergen shows a wheal response which is more than half a centimetre larger than the control, this is considered to indicate an allergy reaction. The control should show less than a one-centimetre wheal, otherwise the test is invalid.

The size of the skin test is believed, by doctors who use this method, to correlate with the severity of clinical symptoms. Critics of this method would argue this is far from the case (see below).

Concurrent use of antihistamine drugs is known to inhibit the response to skin testing.

SPECIFIC IMMUNISATION THERAPY

As early as 1908, Schofield reported in the *Lancet* how he was able to desensitise a boy allergic to egg by administering increasing daily doses over a period of several months.[2] The individual doses were of course extremely small, being the equivalent of one egg in total during six months!

In fact the idea was far from new. King Mithridates VI Eupator, King of Pontus in Asia Minor in the first century BC, took small doses of poisons daily to build up his resistance to them. Evidently the idea worked and he survived several attempts to poison him. He gave us the word mithridate.

A more up-to-date example, now alas familiar to many, is the fact that drug addicts learn to tolerate enormous doses of the substances to which they are addicted, amounts which would quite literally have killed anyone who had not been conditioned to it.

After the discovery that allergenic substances may announce themselves by causing reactions in the skin and thus be identified, specific desensitisation as a treatment for hay-fever, using the information gained from testing the patient, became widely practised. A pioneer in this field was Leonard Noon working in 1911, who used the eye as a site for testing substances, a positive reaction being redness and lachrymation.[3] He showed that steadily increasing doses of the discovered allergens, given as a series of injections prior to the time of year when trouble was expected, occasionally brought relief.

A number of patients become seriously ill with this approach and it has to be discontinued. Still more are not helped at all; the technique is dependent on the accuracy with which the antigens are identified in the initial testing and, as discussed below, this is not high. However it does sometimes work successfully and since for many years it was the only available treatment, it has rightly had its place in the medical armoury.

CRITICISMS OF CONVENTIONAL SKIN TESTING

Clinical ecologists, who are largely indifferent to the immunological approach to maladaptation syndrome, are uniformly critical of this approach. Lawrence Dickey, former president of the American Society for Clinical Ecology, points out that immunologists have made no significant advance in this technique since Noon and Freeman in 1911.

One of the principal points of contention is that foods rarely react using this technique, probably one of the reasons that the belief that food allergies don't exist still persists among doctors. Randolph, Rinkel and Zeller reported that: 'It is our finding that only two patients out of a hundred will give positive skin tests to every food which is allergic.'[4] By allergic foods they meant those which had been clearly demonstrated to make the patient ill by actual feeding tests. Even Feingold, himself an immunologist, admits: 'It is generally recognized that skin testing for foods is unreliable'.[5]

This drawback has been substantiated yet again recently. The very elegant study carried out on eighty-eight migraine child patients at the Great Ormond Street Hospital in 1983 found a similar lack of useful correlation between the results of skin prick tests and what actually made the patients ill.

Furthermore the prick and intradermal tests are considered unsafe by some practitioners. Feeling bad after testing is quite common but deaths have also occurred. These have usually taken place as a result of anaphylactic shock (anaphylaxis, the opposite of prophylaxis), a profound collapse which takes place rapidly and fatally after the patient has undergone some sort of allergic crisis (this may happen due to natural causes and exposures, not just during medical testing). Such deaths are not common but that is poor solace for the families of victims, who perhaps only wanted to know the cause of a rash or wheeze.

Nevertheless, testing of this sort has continued to be used almost exclusively by conventional allergists with their immunological orientation. Richard Mackarness sums up the *status quo* thus:

> By the late 1930s the majority of allergists had limited their activities to giving skin tests and shots for hay fever, asthma, and urticaria, based on the antigen/antibody theory. Anything which they could

> not explain and treat in those terms they pronounced 'not allergic' . . . this attitude – not unconnected with the high profit margins on shots – left a lot of people dissatisfied.[6]

Cynical words from a well-known clinical ecologist. (Remember that allergy-based medical practice, not necessarily the same as the science of allergy, has its largest representation in the USA, where doctors have a financial interest in what treatments are recommended.)

CO-SEASONAL THERAPY

The desensitising technique described above is based on forcing the body to confront bigger and bigger challenges with substances that are hostile to it. It was found to be far safer to do this *prior* to the expected time of trouble. Thus for hay-fever the late winter was considered ideal for a course of treatments. The rationale traditionally has been to peak at the maximum dose just before symptoms would otherwise have developed. Thus the name pre-seasonal therapy suggests itself.

A different technique, which was developed simultaneously and seems to have been largely forgotten except by the clinical ecologists, is to administer the desensitising doses *at the height of the trouble*. This is called co-seasonal therapy and has certain advantages:

1. To begin with, the doses required are much smaller, perhaps comparable with the first challenge of the pre-seasonal method. This increases the safety element greatly.
2. There is no question of missing the optimum time and having to tell the patient to come back in twelve months.
3. Dosing is usually, though not necessarily, on a daily basis and thus the patient has more direct control over the severity of his symptoms. Dosing can be increased as the effects get worse, to bring things quickly under control again. (Self-administration by the patient is actually the norm, rather than being unusual.)

SERIAL TITRATION

Co-seasonal therapy, as described by Vaughan[7] and Hansel[8] was used successfully for many years. A great improvement came with the development of serial titration by Rinkel, arguably the greatest of clinical ecologists to date.

His idea was to ascertain the optimum dose to use in co-seasonal therapy by measuring the efficacy of different strengths in actual usage. Instead of using the traditional 1:10 series of dilutions, he used 1:5 increments, to enable him to verify the most effective dilution much more critically. He defined the optimum dose as 'the one which gives the most complete degree of relief. The period of relief may vary from 3 to 21 days... This dose will vary in different antigens and different patients'.[9]

This enables a safe dose to be worked out for each individual, in accordance with his own personal allergens and susceptibility to them. In practice it takes a certain amount of skill and judgement for the practitioner to arrive at the correct dose. Increasing increments of dilutions of the antigen are administered at two to five day intervals until the relief lasts five days or longer. After that the dose is repeated at the set intervals as a 'maintenance' dose.

For many years this technique was a great advance in the treatment of allergies and its development stood as a milestone. Nevertheless, few doctors ever heard of it. Only a handful of clinical ecologists took an interest.

Even today, it is used occasionally by practising clinical ecologists as a standby. I myself, if I am encountering any difficulties in the implementation of the next method discussed below, which I use extensively, often give patients a series of antigen dilutions and have them determine which one works best by therapeutic trial; a crude but effective method of 'titration'!

THE PROVOCATION-NEUTRALISATION TECHNIQUE

Carleton Lee in Missouri, in the late 1950s, came up with yet another improvement on the dilution approach. As so often happens in science, his discovery followed on a chance observation. Events must occur many times and in many places which have profound scientific importance and pass unnoticed. It is unlikely that Alexander Fleming was the first man ever to see bacteria on a culture plate destroyed by a contaminating mould, but he was certainly the first to realise the significance of what he saw. It is only when the right man, with the acumen and knowledge to judge the usefulness of an observation, is in the right place at the right time that we have a startling new discovery. Thus Fleming discovered Penicillin and Carleton Lee invented the provocation-neutralisation technique.

Lee was experimenting by injecting varying dilutions of antigens and he noticed two things. Firstly, patients occasionally felt ill as a result, which wasn't surprising, since he was using potential allergens. But what did amaze him was that they occasionally felt suddenly well. It seemed that at times a particular dilution, when injected, would relieve symptoms within minutes. Further trials showed this to be a very effective way of determining Rinkel's 'optimal dose'. The method was really a serial end-point skin titration technique but is known usually as provocation-neutralisation procedure. This comes from the fact that symptoms are first provoked and then switched off or neutralised.

Over the years it has been widely used and is very successful – in the right hands. This rider has to be added because, like many techniques in and out of medicine, if it is done haphazardly it won't work or may even make the situation worse. It has also been found to be effective against both food allergens, inhaled substances (such as dust and mould) and, rather surprisingly, even chemicals such as petrol fumes and formaldehyde.

The definitive text on this revolutionary approach to dealing with allergies is by Dr Joseph Miller. He includes a personal historical note in his book:

> After following conventional methods for thirteen years, I heard Carleton H. Lee deliver a paper on provocative testing in 1965, at a meeting of the American College of Allergists in Chicago.
>
> I was naturally skeptical [sic], but tried his suggestions when I returned to my office. The results can only be described as astounding. Many patients with unresolved allergic problems responded markedly and rapidly. Many with resistant asthma or perennial allergic rhinitis improved greatly or cleared completely when food injection therapy was added to their inhalant injection therapy. Some patients whose asthma or rhinitis was well controlled by inhalant therapy obtained remarkable relief of other types of symptoms, such as headache, vertigo, laryngeal oedema, spastic colon, chronic urticaria, learning problems, and extrasytoles when food injection therapy was added.

I gradually found myself successfully treating and relieving not just the half-dozen clinical entities normally seen in allergy practise but fifty or more formerly refractory symptoms and syndromes.[10]

The technique is now often known, ironically, as the Miller Method rather than being named after Lee. It is worth describing in detail as it will undoubtedly become more widely used as time goes by.

The clinic will have on hand a large battery of available tests, to suit the clinical condition of varying patients and their presenting symptoms. It is usual to arrange the most concentrated solution to be one per cent, though this is by no means mandatory. Stronger doses can provoke quite severe symptoms at times. Incidentally, the extracts used must be of the very highest purity; thus, for example, the foodstuffs extracts will have been grown without any chemical treatments such as weed-killer. A few commercial companies make these specially for use by allergists.

The most concentrated test solution will be labelled No. 1. In addition there are also a series of dilutions of the same allergen following on, 2,3,4 etc., to at least No. 9. Each increment is 1:5 of the previous solution. Owing to the power of exponential numbers, these dilutions become very large, as the table below will show.

Some substances, eg. the house-dust mite, would be too potent to use with a starting strength of 1 per cent. For safety

TABLE 5.1 RELATIVE DILUTIONS USED IN PROVOCATION-NEUTRALISATION TECHNIQUES

Solution	*Dilution*
1 (1%)	1:100
2	1:500
3	1:2500
4	1:12,500
5	1:62,500
6	1:312,500
7	1:1,562,500
8	1:7,812,500
9	1:39,062,500

reasons, the No. 1 dose is usually arranged at 0.1 per cent. Even then the reactions are occasionally severe but thanks to being able to neutralise the effect rapidly, the patient isn't distressed for long.

METHOD

The physician injects a small dose of the weakest solution, say No 9, on the outer part of the upper arm. This amount is usually 0.05 millilitre, sufficient to creat a wheal approximately four millimetres in diameter. After ten minutes the wheal is read and the patient questioned for any symptoms which may have arisen as a result of the injection.

If the wheal has grown two millimetres or more this is good evidence of an allergic reaction. Additional positive signs include blanching, induration and a sharp edge to the wheal. If most or all of these signs are absent, the wheal is considered negative and this is a sign of a dose that is probably too weak or an 'underdose' as Miller refers to it. The patient may or may not have symptoms. A wheal with most of the above signs is considered positive or an 'overdose'. Once again, the patient may or may not have symptoms.

The judgement of the clinician comes in when it comes to deciding to interpret the findings. If the wheal is negative but the patient has symptoms, this is a definite allergen. He wants then to locate the probable neutralising dose. If he is underdosing he wants to go stronger to arrive at the neutralising dose, i.e. injecting decreasing numbers, such as 8,7,6 and so on.

He should arrive at a point where the symptoms disappear and the wheal is negative. If he then continues to go stronger still the wheal begins to manifest signs of overdosing. The symptoms may return. The first negative wheal, without symptoms, that precedes the overdosing effect is taken to be the neutralising dose.

Does all this sound complicated? Well it is. There is quite a degree of skill involved in deciding exactly where the end-point lies. There are many variables and strange manifestations that may occur to make it even more confusing. But throughout all, a neutralising dose remains one which has no symptoms at the end of ten minutes and a negative wheal. Usually only one dilution has these characteristics and in the majority of tests this is quite straightforward.

THE 'ENGLISH METHOD'

A variation of the above technique described by Miller I think of as the English version. This is because it is used exclusively by those English ecologists who use the provocation-neutralisation method, though in fact it was developed in the USA and introduced here by Mackarness in the late 1970s. It is described briefly in Miller's book.

The difference is to start with strong doses of the allergen being tested and working towards weaker solutions. We abandon the standard of four millimetre starting wheal and inject 0.1 millilitres of test solution, making the largest possible wheal (about 10mm × 10mm is ideal).

If this grows in ten minutes by two millimetres or more and/or symptoms are present, this is treated as a positive result. The next weaker solution is then used. If the initial wheal grew by a substantial amount the No. 2 could not be an end-point and it is justifiable to skip to, say, No. 3 or even No. 4. The characteristics of the neutralising dose however remain exactly the same, namely a wheal which exibits no growth, hardness, blanching or sharp edge, when no symptom is present. It is permissible for a symptom to come on briefly during the administration of a neutralising dose, providing that it has completely cleared again after ten minutes. This is easy to illustrate and the diagram shows a typical sequence of events leading up to the end-point (Fig. 6).

Passing beyond the neutralising dose often leads to the patient developing symptoms. This is the underdosing band described by Miller. The wheal may also resume a growth characteristic. Ironically, underdosing symptoms are often more unpleasant than those caused by overdosing.

Starting with the most concentrated solutions, provoked symptoms are much less commonly encountered than in the weak-to-strong method. Therefore the patient has an easier time of it. A number of false negatives may be encountered because the starting dose lies near to the end-point and little growth takes place and no symptom is reported. This is easily overcome, if the physician suspects a substance because of the patient's history,

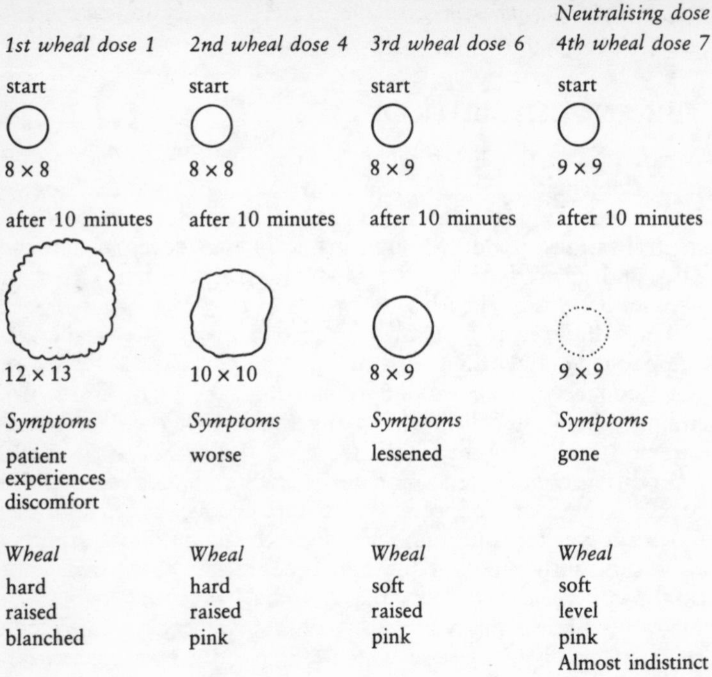

(The size of the wheal at start is immaterial)

Fig. 6 *Wheal responses in Miller's method*

by going more dilute before declaring it not an allergy. If nothing happens on a No. 1, the No. 3 may well cause symptoms and perhaps even exhibit growth.

The great advantage of the provocation–neutralisation technique over conventional skin testing methods is that it yields information about which substances cause symptoms in that particular patient. Allergens are injected one at a time, instead of a dozen or more at a time; thus a symptom is highly significant. Bearing in mind that the absolute doses are very small indeed, compared to actual ingestion of the food, any substance which causes a symptom at this level must be a notable allergen.

Conventional allergists to whom I have shown this technique are all startled by the frequency with which symptoms can be provoked, especially in regard to foods, which rarely show any sign of reaction using the prick test. When asked, I can give no satisfactory explanation for this but I feel there are two probable factors: allergens behave differently when given singly as opposed to many at once, and the higher starting doses differ from the normal strength of prick test solutions which are equivalent to about No. 3 or No. 4 strength in Miller's method. Many of these would therefore be in the end-point zone, if not actually end-points, and yield false negative results.

Using the neutralising method, knowing that it is simple to 'switch off' any reaction provoked, the clinical ecologist can quite confidently use a No. 1 solution which is one per cent. This would be dangerous in the prick test, as the patient has no protection against serious after-effects, including anaphylactic shock. Of course this does not explain why much more *dilute* doses, in the first method, should also provoke symptoms almost routinely.

CONTROVERSY

Clinical ecology as a whole could not be said to be anything but controversial in the medical profession. The discord however seems to reach its acme in the bitter and acrimonious debate about the effectiveness of the neutralising dose method. I myself have used it for many years and am more than satisfied with its workability but of course that is nothing more than my opinion.

The usual criticism from orthodox colleagues is that it is unproven scientifically and they point out gleefully that nothing definitive has been written in medical literature of the appropriate standing.

The actual truth is that many good scientific studies have been done over the years, meeting all normal criteria for validity and yet *no journal will publish them.* Dr Marvin Boris of New York for example carried out a simple but convincing double-blind cross-over trial demonstrating that neutralising drops protected asthmatic patients against the effects of animal hair and danders. But it has yet to see the light of day in print. Probably it never will, except in minor journals with editorial freedom not dominated by the finances of drug company cartels (need I say more?).

More recently, Dr Jonathan Brostoff, a senior consultant in immunology at the Middlesex and, incidentally, a much respected clinical ecologist, has also obtained convincing proof. His scientific pedigree is impeccable but it remains to be seen whether his work will be accepted by journals such as the *Lancet* or *British Medical Journal.*

Suppressing truth and knowledge is always a sad and degrading business for such a glorious thinking creature as Man but nowhere is it so deplorably evil as in the field of healing the sick and hurt. However one message of this book is that such information *is* being suppressed and you had better take steps to acquire it yourself!

SUBLINGUAL TESTING

An interesting related technique to serial skin titration is to use the sublingual (under the tongue) route of administration. For certain groups of patients, notably children, this has the advantage of being less distressing than intracutaneous injections every ten minutes over the space of some hours.

There is no essential difference in this approach but naturally there are fewer parameters by which to judge reactions or lack of them. Instead of being able to view a wheal and its size and characteristics the clinician has only the patient's subjective symptoms to rely upon, plus what he can observe for himself objectively. In fact, with practice, it is possible to become quite adept at spotting subtle shifts in mood or attitude, restlessness, skin colour etc. The neutralising dose would be that at which the patient reports his symptoms have switched off and the clinician sees that whatever manifestations were turned on have disappeared again.

The serial dilutions may be made 1:10 or 1:5 according to preference. The size of the dose used in testing is said to be immaterial but usually 0.1 millilitre is preferred. Lawrence Dickey, a former surgeon, now retired and practising clinical ecology exclusively for many years, and incidentally one of clinical ecology's gifted writers, has the following observations to make about his use of the technique:

> Sublingual clinical titration is the other method we use to arrive at a safe, effective sublingual dosage. It is our modification of the provocative food test originally described by Rinkel *et al* [see chapter 4]. Symptoms are either present or induced by:
>
> 1. deliberate feeding test;

2. inhalation testing;
   (a) particulates (e.g. pollen and mold spores) by sniff;
   (b) gaseous emissions from liquid, etc. kept in a closed jar;
3. intracutaneous provocation;
4. subcutaneous provocation;
5. sublingual provocation.

We have used all of the above methods except the subcutaneous. This method is used by Willoughby and others. We use the intracutaneous method first, following the technique originally described by Rinkel *et al.* Since 1963, after learning the sublingual technique from Pfeiffer, we have used it extensively. The first two methods are used occasionally.

In provoking symptoms we usually start with the number 1. dilution except when the history indicates a high degree of susceptibility, in which case we start with a weaker dilution. If there are no symptoms with a No. 1 dilution we proceed to a No. 3 dilution and occasionally to a No. 5 if we suspect the patient is sensitive. This is because the stronger dilutions are often neutralising, and symptoms may be produced with a weaker dilution and then neutralised by trying the strong solutions again. This phenomenon of provoking symptoms with a weak solution and then relieving them with a stronger one was noted by Lee. This seems paradoxical but has proven to be a common experience to those performing this type of testing. This is why we are not content with drawing conclusions from tests using a single dilution.

The neutralising or turn-off dose is a weaker or stronger 1:5 dilution than that which induced the reaction. We have termed this clinical titration because we are guided by symptom response rather than skin whealing.[11]

The paper is available in full, as a useful booklet for practitioners, from Action Against Allergy, 43, The Downs, London SW20 8HG.

Dickey admits to a few experiences he terms 'adventures' and 'misadventures' with a candour rare among fellows of the so-called 'scientific' medical fraternity.

First for the misadventures. We have had the patients use the drops accidentally in the place of nose drops, drink part of the bottle or ingest it when the bottle spilled on a sandwich in a lunch pail. The reactions were only temporarily distressing. The patient who used them as nose drops said he became a little dizzy but they cleared his nose. There have been some brisk reactions in petrochemical testing, but we have never had a reaction in testing or treatment that was at all life-threatening.

> As to the adventures, we have been especially gratified by the prompt relief of presenting symptoms obtained with serial-dilution titration testing, using one allergen at a time which history indicated to be involved. Treatment using these relieving doses has been quite effective. Using the method of testing one allergen at a time has made it possible to salvage some patients who were not doing well and to detemine the truly essential specific components of their prescription.

He then goes on to say:

> Patients, by varying their dosage, determine their own optimal dose, and over a period of time most of them reduce their frequency of dosage. Many are able to discontinue their drops when they have controlled some of the dietary and other environmental factors that were adversely affecting them. One patient had a dust and mold prescription that was quite effective, and then went an entire year without taking it but resumed taking the same prescription, with relief, a year later. This experience, along with others, indicated that the effectiveness of the prescription did not deteriorate with time, as we had assumed.

Finally, he makes an important point which is reiterated by other clinical ecologists and should not be lost sight of; that in the management of food allergy, the primary emphasis should be on avoidance, rotation and diversification of the diet, with sublingual therapy used only when rotation and avoidance are impossible.

The main benefit of the sub-lingual 'drops' therapy is that it enables patients occasionally to eat foods they otherwise could not, and so allows them to lead relatively normal lives without being dietary 'freaks'.

6

Further Testing Methods

We next come to review a number of alternative methods of diagnosing allergies; that is, other than food challenge tests or skin testing. The wide diversity of these approaches is perhaps a reflection of the complexity and far-reaching consequences of allergies or hypersensitivities, which distort or disrupt a number of different body systems.

These are not listed in any deliberate order of preference or reliability.

CYTOTOXIC TESTING

Tests which depend on the agglutination or disruption of blood cells have been known for many years. For example Rose and Waaler showed that sheep blood cells may be agglutinated in a significant number of cases by serum taken from rheumatoid arthritis sufferers.

Basically these tests are designed to elicit the presence of antibodies to the substance being questioned. If such antibodies are present, a reaction takes place which clumps or weakens the cells involved in the preparation. It does not matter, in terms of the accuracy of the test, what these antibodies are due to. Food antibodies may be detected just like any other. White cells may be used conveniently for detection of antibodies to food substances: the so-called cytotoxic test.

Today's test follows thirty years of refinement. Use of this sort of reaction for *in vitro* screening for food allergy antibodies was first recorded by P. Black in 1956. The test at that time was crude and produced results which were best described as suggestive, rather than conclusive. It pointed the way, however.

Since 1960 the test has been steadily researched and refined by W. T. K. and M. P. Bryan at the Washington University School of Medicine, St Louis, Missouri. The technique is simple but depends for accuracy upon a high standard of laboratory technique. Microscope slides are coated with a silicone compound and three petroleum jelly rings are extruded into each slide. Into each ring is inserted a known quantity of food extract and the slides are dried in a dust-free environment.

Ten millilitres of fresh venous blood is citrated (at the time of collection, to stop it clotting) and centrifuged at the laboratory. The buffy coat (one of the layers, containing white cells and platelets) is drawn off, remixed with serum and sterile water, a quantity placed within each petroleum jelly ring on the slides and the chamber sealed with a cover slip.

The slides are observed at intervals over the next two hours, using a × 60 magnification dry lens. Although effects on the red cells and platelets are noted, the most important effect is that on the white cells, especially the neutrophils.

Healthy neutrophils are mobile and exhibit ameoboid behaviour. Granules in the cytoplasm stream freely and pseudopodia are formed and re-formed constantly.

On contact with allergens, in this case food samples, the cells lose their mobility, cease to form pseudopodia and become rounded in shape. The cytoplasmic granules become sluggish and cease to stream. Eventually, damaged cells vacuolate, rupture and die.

It is customary to grade reactions from 0 to 4, depending on severity of damage, observing the following changes:

(a) reduction or loss of pseudopodia and amoeboid movement;
(b) intracellular stasis;
(c) rounding and distortion of cell contour;
(d) vacuolation;
(e) cell lysis.

Dr Damien Downing, medical director of the York Medical and Nutritional Laboratory, which carries out cytotoxic testing, naturally believes it to be an effective and reliable method. He claims the test has an eighty per cent accuracy and, whatever its shortcomings, it is, he says, the quickest and most effective way for practitioners to identify their patients' allergies.

The difficulty with the test, in common with many others, is that it rests in the final analysis on human interpretation, rather than measurement. This isn't so bad, as long as each laboratory is at least consistent with its own standards. But it may, on occasion, lead to patchy quality in results which serve the patient ill. It's one thing to be told you're allergic to something when you are not. But the reverse, to be told you are not allergic to something when you are may completely deny recovery.

Something of a stir was created in the media recently when a national newspaper sent two identical specimens to the same laboratory for cytotoxic testing, using a different name for each. The results for the two samples were so at variance as to throw doubt on the entire method. The report carried the obvious innuendo that the laboratory centre in question was out to make money at the expense of a gullible public and its scientific standards did not justify faith in its methods. Incidentally, I should make it clear that the York laboratory was *not* the one in question.

In actual fact, these inconsistencies, the stuff of newspaper drama, need not concern us unduly. Dr Downing comments on the reproducibility of the test:

> If the same blood is examined in two separate preparations simultaneously, or in the same preparation by two technicians, or the same blood is examined at 24-hour intervals under controlled conditions, with any single increase in the degrees of freedom one generally finds that between one in five and one in six of the test results cross the border from one to another of the four possible results. This is presumably a reflection of the technicians' human limitations. Greater degrees of variability are rare, at around one per cent. That is to say that a technician can manage to get the result accurate to within one degree of reaction 99 per cent of the time![1]

This sounds almost too good to be true, until you remember that in this case each one 'degree' of reaction represents twenty-five per cent of the whole!

Another major source of inaccuracy is that the specimen must be as fresh as possible. As soon as the blood leaves the body it begins to deteriorate. It may remain viable for up to twenty-four hours after collection; enough for success if transit through the postal system is rapid but not if it is delayed for any reason.

One of the problems in deciding on the accuracy of the tests is what to use as a comparison. For practical reasons, though not theoretically sound, it is customary to rely on the results of food elimination and challenge tests, as described in Chapter 4. In other words, if the food causes symptoms on a properly carried out challenge test it is an allergen, if it doesn't, it is not. Ideally, double-blind challenges would be used, to avoid psychologically induced false positives. But there is no way of ruling out false negatives which, as every clinical ecologist knows, are quite common after just one or two test feeds.

However, the fact remains that what counts is workability and not scientific demonstrable accuracy, i.e. does the patient get well using the data from such a test? In regard to this point, it is worth considering the results of a California 1981 study.[2] This was intended to investigate the cytotoxic test from the immunological point of view and showed there was every likelihood of a 'conventional' immunological mechanism (see Chapter 2) for the cytotoxic phenomenon. The experimenter performed the cytotoxic test on sixty-five subjects and used this as a basis to select allergens. For the test group he used cytotoxic positive foods and for the control group cytotoxic negative foods. All patients thought they had cytotoxic positive foods.

They were told to eat this food regularly for several weeks, then to eliminate it for five days, and on the fifth day to eat it again, beginning at breakfast. Blood specimens were taken before the elimination, to obtain baselines, and again at 8 a.m. and 6 p.m. on the day of challenge.

What interests us here is that, out of the test group of fifty-five, fifty-three developed symptoms after the challenge, ranging from irritability, restlessness and insomnia, to severe symptoms including laryngeal odoema. None of the controls developed symptoms. It is somewhat facile to say that the cytotoxic negative foods were 100 per cent accurate and the cytotoxic positive ones at least 95 per cent correct but essentially that is what these coincidental results implied.

Probably the main drawback of the cytotoxic test method is

that it needs intelligent and knowledgeable back-up by a competent doctor. Otherwise the patient may get himself on to strange and inadequate diets by avoidance of the positive foods. Unfortunately, this back-up is not always readily obtainable and the laboratories themselves often duck this issue. At the time of writing, in the UK there is only one such laboratory run by a qualified medical doctor and that is the one at York referred to above.

I do not share Dr Downing's view that this is the best method. He compares it favourably with other immunological tests, such as the RAST test (see below) and conventional skin testing. However he discreetly avoids mention of Miller's provocation-neutralisation technique, which I prefer. I think it is better for two reasons. Firstly, the patient does not usually need to avoid a food found positive but merely to eat it in moderation using neutralising drops. Thus the need for strange and restricting diets is less. Secondly, the patient gets a very good subjective reality on his allergens due to the symptoms caused by the provocation nature of Miller's method. Nothing impresses on a patient's mind the nature of his illness more than feeling ill due to a known reaction. (It must be pointed out that not all patients experience pronounced symptoms with this technique.)

As against this, however, the Miller method has nothing to offer the patient who is forced to go it alone. Whereas cytotoxic testing can be of great help to an intelligent individual who is prepared to read up the nature of allergies, if he has no other available medical assistance (which is all too often the case).

COMPREHENSIVE ENVIRONMENTAL CONTROL UNITS

Allergies never come alone. Susceptible individuals who develop a reaction to one substance are quite likely to do the same for others. The purely food allergic individual probably does not exist though, as I commented in Chapter 4, it is possible to make many patients well simply by attention to their food allergens, because foods form the bulk of substances with which we come into intimate contact.

The fact is that most patients react also to so-called environmental factors, such as atmospheric pollution, dusts, moulds and chemicals at home and work. Some are so badly affected that they may never recover through dietary management alone.

Still fewer are so bad that they improve only very slightly under conditions normally available to them. Except with those who are frightened of their affliction (most are not), it is possible to joke with the patient that they should ideally live on a desert island in the middle of the ocean. Clearly this is impossible. But there is a serious side to this irony. What if it were possible to construct an oasis where such people could retreat and escape from the hostilities of their environment? Would such an artificial environment have any diagnostic use?

Dr Theron Randolph of Chicago decided it would. He began to experiment in the late 1950s with a comprehensive environmental control programme. This involves keeping the patient in special quarters, a so-called ecology unit, shielded from everyday contacts. The air is supplied filtered and chemically 'clean'. Only spring water is permitted. Special nursing procedures are used to avoid such common but potentially adverse encounters as felt-tip pens, scents, detergents and even plastic waste-paper bins. The wall coverings have to be of neutral materials. Beds and other furnishings are metal or wood, floors are left untreated, linen is cotton or otherwise natural fibre. Foam rubber is also banned, which precludes carpeting, synthetic pillows and upholstered chairs etc. Even televisions are banned; they give off hot plastic fumes when in use. Cosmetics are not allowed, either for the nursing staff or inmates, and all personal effects which would inhibit the success of the programme are removed. In other words the cleanest possible environment is provided, free of all avoidable chemical contamination.

On entering the unit the patient is put on a fast, to ensure that simultaneously they cut out their food allergens. Nature does the rest. Depending on the condition of the patient, he or she may begin to improve within a few hours. Certainly recovery should take place within five days, the time it takes for the bowel to clear of offending foods. This is usually speeded up with a mild purge. Drugs are discontinued immediately if it is safe to do so and in all cases within a short time. It is remarkable how these medications prove to be non-essential once the patient is in safe surroundings.

As with all unmasking procedures, withdrawal symptoms are the rule rather than the exception. These may be very severe but the patient has the comfort of knowing he or she is surrounded by skilled staff who understand and are familiar with the problem. These effects eventually abate and the patient is then on the road to recovery, often for the first time in many years.

Naturally, if the patient does not recover it is possible to say with some conviction that his or her illness is not allergy-based. However with skilled selection procedures this rarely if ever happens. For the well-chosen patient indeed it is magical relief and provides the dramatic much-needed confirmation that there is nothing *intrinsically* wrong with the patient but that the illness has an exogenous cause. It is rather an extreme approach but for most sufferers any amount of effort is worthwhile if it gets to the bottom of their condition.

The next step comes in breaking the fast. Only the purest chemically un-contaminated foods must be used, beginning with unusual foods, as described in chapter 4. Next come foods eaten every three days or more often, with the expectation of some reactions. If symptoms are provoked, neutral foods may be continued but all new tests are discontinued until the symptoms have cleared. Finally, come dairy, wheat and corn, the worst offenders. Randolph has these tested at two consecutive meals, taking no chances that an allergy to these major offenders will be missed. The pulse rate is counted before and after the test meal (see Coca's pulse method below). Reactions are usually quite quick. Randolph says:

> Clinically detectable evidence of a reaction to a food formerly eaten regularly and frequently but avoided completely for four to ten days prior to that test feeding is usually noted by the experienced observer within the first hour. There are two phases of the test reaction. The first phase may be so mild in character and so transient in duration as to be missed. This is commonly followed by a relative improvement for several hours prior to the more apparent delayed reaction.[3]

As against this however, some cases, who are perhaps less sensitive, may need two or three days of cumulative ingestion of foods before evidencing a convincing reaction. How does the clinician know which these cases are? He doesn't, at least not in advance. Therefore considerable skill and judgement is sometimes required to get each patient through this stage of the challenges.

Next come chemicals. It is prudent to allow the patient to try the normally commercially available foods which may be contaminated with fungicides, sulphur, waxes and other agents, as part of his challenges. If he can tolerate at least some, so much the better. Obtaining chemically un-contaminated foods is difficult and expensive, especially in the UK, where clinical ecology is not as widely comprehended as in the USA.

Finally, a number of commonly occurring chemical contacts can be studied by exposing the patient to test doses of them. Such substances would include household gas, formaldehyde, synthetic alcohols, fresh newspapers and perhaps cigarette smoke and other likely allergens, depending on the judgement of the clinician in charge of the case.

When all this is over and the patient is well he may then return home. This brings new challenges, deliberately or inadvertently, which in turn provide more information. During this time the patient must maintain his ideal safe diet, as worked out in the unit, re-exposing himself a little at a time to facets of his regular environment. In fact this is often a very trying time for the patient, who may find himself being made repeatedly ill due to all kinds of unsuspected agents such as mould and danders, carpet treatments, synthetic fabrics, cooking smells etc. This is the principal criticism I have heard expressed, even by clinical ecologists, of this otherwise logical holistic approach.

Ideally, he or she would start with an empty home and only allow in those items which fail to provoke a response. In practice it is necessary to work the other way round and gradually identify and remove offending items from the home. This may not be easy, bearing in mind the average modern home is totally unsuited to the ecology patient (see chapter 10).

The question sometimes arises of the safety of such drastic procedures. Randolph comments:

> Initial complete food deprivation is a safe procedure as judged by the absence of complication in fasting over 5,000 patients ranging in age between one and eighty years. Neither are there any untoward reactions following initial feedings, providing compatible foods are fed.[4]

In regard to chemical testing he is rather more cautious: 'the deliberate exposure of patients to measured doses of given chemicals may be hazardous in view of the extreme range of susceptibility that may be involved'.[5]

He goes on to point out however that there are ways chemicals may be diluted and tested safely.

Naturally units such as these are expensive to run and consequently the fees very high indeed. In the USA, where the alternative is years of costly and largely ineffective conventional therapy, the patients may consider a spell in an ecology unit a relatively good investment, just in terms of finance, never mind well-being. In the UK, with a free health service, this may not be so clear.

The first such unit to be opened here is that under the charge of Dr Jonathan Maberley, a consultant physician at the Airedale hospital in Yorkshire. His ecology unit, opened in 1985, is available only for private patients and with fees of several hundreds of pounds a week it seems likely that, apart from those with fairly substantial personal means, only those lucky enough to be part of a private health insurance scheme before the onset of their illness will be able to afford to go.

Nevertheless, it is an exciting new development and he will undoubtedly have more clientele than he can cope with, at least until other such units are made available. So far, Dr Maberley's is the only one of its kind in Europe.

THE PULSE METHOD

Dr Arthur Coca, a leading American allergist, states that his wife first reported that her pulse raced after eating certain foods. On that simple observation this great pioneer doctor, one who comfortably bridged the gap between clinical ecology and conventional immunologically oriented allergy work, was able to build a very interesting technique for detecting allergies, especially to foods. Because he clearly identified a group of patients who had food allergies, it ran in families and no antibodies or other humoral agents were ever found to explain the reaction (or yet have been), he called it familial non-reaginic food-allergy. A further characteristic of this type of allergy reaction is that it frequently raises the pulse rate.

He coined the word idioblapsis (life-spoiler) for this manifestation but it has not been generally accepted. Nevertheless, it is a very widespread phenomenon in the population; Coca puts it as high as ninety per cent on circumstantial evidence. Indeed the theme of this book is that most people have some degree of this problem, whether it is making them ill at present or not.

Coca explains the basis of his discovery:

> the heart is one of the most dependable, human, physiological constants. In the present connection its significant characters are the following two:
> (a) The daily range from low to high is rarely greater than 16 beats per minute.
> (b) The daily maximum does not vary more than two beats per minute.
>
> If, then, the daily range of the pulse exceeds 20 and the daily maximal counts per minute vary more than two beats, the patient is practically certainly affected with idioblaptic allergy. If, furthermore, the maximal count is 88 or higher, this is corroborative evidence, and the diagnosis can be upheld.[6]

It must be pointed out that this refers to a *resting* pulse and that there must be no other manifest clinical condition which would account for a high or variable pulse rate, such as a fever, heart disease, thyroid excess, anaemia etc.

He goes on to say: 'Rarely the food allergic patient may present a completely normal pulse-record for several days on an unrestricted diet – a somewhat disturbing experience when first encountered.'

He need not have been concerned about this apparent contradiction to his technique. In those days he did not know, as we do now, about the hidden or masked allergy effect which explains why a patient may eat or drink hostile foods without any *apparent* effect whatsoever.

Coca's method has two aspects. Firstly, he advocates a charted survey of the pulse over several days, taking the pulse before rising, before and twice after each meal and then on retiring. This record may then be studied in the light of the above criteria. The chart we use in my own clinic is shown as Table 6.1. This particular example comes from a 55-year-old lady with arthritis. It shows a range of twenty-eight beats. Also you may note that each time she ate banana the pulse rate increased sharply and this did indeed turn out to be one of her allergies. However, so were tea, milk, egg and beef but these caused no reaction on this survey, presumably due to the masking effect.

It is difficult to identify specific allergens by means of this chart. The example just given illustrates this clearly. It serves only as a general guide to the case. If by chance, however, it shows periods of normal pulse rate (such as on Day 1 and Day

6 in Table 6.1), the foods eaten before these periods may be selected as 'safe' and if the patient concentrates on those foods, he or she may then have a steady base-line upon which to project individual feeding tests, that is to say a pulse which behaves itself, except when reacting to allergens under test.

Individual food tests Coca carries out on the basis of five small meals a day, consisting of one single food to be tested at each sitting. He recommends small portions, so that the reaction, if there is one, clears more quickly. This may be contrasted with my recommendations on page 83 (Chapter 4). The resting pulse is used and it must be counted for a full minute. It is recorded before ingesting the food and again thirty, sixty and ninety minutes afterwards. Naturally the patient should avoid any provocative activities in the interim, otherwise confusion may occur, though it is not necessary to sit still for the entire one and a half hours.

Safe foods may be used cumulatively. That is, foods which do not demonstrably raise the pulse may be eaten along with the new food under test. The time of day and also the sequence in which foods are tested is unimportant, he stated, though today we benefit by being able to suggest avoiding foods from the same family within the same two-day period, in case inadvertent cross-reaction and masking occurs.

Essentially it is a simple method and can easily be carried out by the individual on him or her self. However there are one or two pitfalls, other than those mentioned above in passing. For example cumulative reactions can occur. That is a food has little or no effect at first but as it is eaten repeatedly as a 'safe' food it steadily increases the pulse rate. This can usually be sorted out by rotating safe foods.

Environmental factors may also confuse the issue. It may appear that a food is causing a reaction when in fact it was due to something in the room at the time of testing. It is important to keep conditions as static as possible, to avoid this difficulty.

He gives a special compressed test for tobacco sensitivity, as follows:

> Before beginning to smoke the patient counts his pulse twice at five to ten minute intervals making sure that the rate is within his normal range; after the first puff he makes five counts at three minute intervals. If the rate at any of these counts rises above his *normal* maximum he (she) is to be considered allergic to tobacco.[7]

TABLE 6.1 ONE-WEEK PULSE SURVEY

	Day 1	*Day 2*	*Day 3*	*Day 4*	*Day 5*	*Day 6*	*Day 7*
pulse before breakfast	72	88	74	78	82	77	80
List food eaten for breakfast here	tea/milk, melon, egg	tea/milk, toast	tea/milk, bacon, egg, toast	tea/milk, apple, banana	tea/milk, smoked haddock, toast, egg	tea/milk, bacon, egg, toast	tea/milk, apple, toast
30 mins after breakfast	74	86	78	93	80	83	76
60 mins after breakfast	80	80	82	85	81	76	76
pulse before lunch	76	70	76	81	74	80	68
List food eaten for lunch here	cheese sandwich, chocolate biscuit, apple juice	ham, tomato, lettuce, banana, tea/milk	nut roast, tomato, lettuce, coleslaw, apple juice	cod in batter, potatoes, tea/milk	roast beef sandwich, orange, tea/milk	ham salad, tea/milk, biscuit	cheese sandwich, banana, ice cream, coffee/milk

pulse 30 mins after lunch	82	72	74	78	78	72	84
60 mins after lunch	72	84	68	84	83	74	82
pulse before dinner	78	76	72	80	74	71	76
List foods eaten for dinner here	steak, potato, broccoli, swede, gravy, cheesecake, coffee/ cream	lamb chop, potatoes, cabbage, pear, cheese/ biscuits, wine	spaghetti bolognese, date and walnut cake, coffee/ cream	roast pork, roast potatoes, cabbage, swede, gravy, coffee/ milk, cake	shepherd's pie, peas, carrots, gravy, tinned pears, cream, coffee	lamb casserole, with onions, carrot, potato, turnip, ice cream, cheese/ biscuits, coffee	chilli con carne, salad, apple pie, cream, coffee
pulse 30 mins after dinner	80	76	74	76	78	65	80
60 mins after dinner	80	78	80	78	76	70	72

He goes on to say that if the count remains within the normal range there is no reason to think smoking is harmful to that individual and he may smoke thereafter, advice which would make today's doctor cringe. There are many ways in which tobacco harms us that are not allergic in mechanism. I would add that we now know the accuracy of the test would be vastly improved by strict avoidance of tobacco for several days before this test, a preliminary which many smokers would find unbearably difficult. (I have many patients who say they will gladly give up cigarettes once they know they are allergic to them; I am forced to say that nobody will know unless they give up smoking first!)

To conclude this section, two examples of specific food testing are shown in tabular form. The first comes from a twelve-year-old girl with migraines; her mother carried out the pulse checks. The second is from a 47-year-old businessman with asthma. Both cases improved dramatically by avoiding the danger foods. Incidentally, the results in both instances were found to correspond very well with what was found on serial end-point skin titration (Miller method).

TABLE 6.2 TWO EXAMPLES OF SPECIFIC FOOD TESTING

Patient A			
food	*before*	*after 20 minutes*	*after 40 minutes*
wheat	76	78	74
milk*	72	84	82
egg*	78	88	92
apple	73	76	70
potato	68	74	73
pork*	71	83	82
cane sugar	74	76	72
beet sugar*	70	83	82
Patient B			
wheat*	72	85	86
tea	68	74	71
coffee	68	72	76
milk	75	82	79
orange	76	80	78
potato*	72	85	78

*Foods which provoked a pulse reaction

ENZYME POTENTIATED DESENSITISATION (EPD)

This procedure may sometimes help patients who do not seem to respond to any other procedures. It was pioneered by Dr Len McEwen, a London clinical ecologist, who has used it for almost two decades. The main drawback is that it is not diagnostic, that is during the course of investigations the patient and physician do not set out to discover the nature of the principal allergens. However, for patients who already know what they react to and especially where this encompasses many different allergens, such as foods, danders, dusts, moulds, spores etc., it offers the possibility of overcoming at least the worst of the resulting effects and of making life tolerable. Even where the main allergens are not known, an attempt can be made to overcome this problem by including as many as possible of the likely major allergens.

A small area of the forearm is scarified with a scalpel and the desensitising fluid is held over this area by means of a small inverted cup taped to the arm for twenty-four hours.

The desensitising fluid contains extremely small doses of allergenic extracts, including those known to be important to the patient but in addition up to six or seven dozen other such substances may be added, where these may be deemed likely culprits.

Mixed with these extracts are several 'potentiators', including – glucuronidase, hyalase, chondroitin and protamine. The latter substances are to ensure tissue penetration. The glucuronidase, in some unknown way, assists the body in gaining tolerance to the allergens to which it is simultaneously exposed; it is present in all parts of the body under normal circumstances but its role in this process is far from clear. Nevertheless, it does seem essential for the effectiveness of the method.

The dosage levels required in EPD are very tiny indeed, far smaller than the quantities of food which appear in the blood after eating a meal. Thus if the process is attempted shortly after eating the foods the results may be impaired. Therefore the patient is asked to avoid those foods to which he or she is allergic. As already pointed out, however, the patient may be unaware of his or her allergens. In this case, the patient is advised either to fast or to eat only a very restricted diet, devised by Dr

McEwen, for a period of forty-eight hours before the desensitising dose and for at least twenty-four hours afterwards.

There are few contra-indications to this therapy but prudence suggests avoiding it during pregnancy, concurrent infections and close to other vaccination attempts (e.g. smallpox, polio or BCG). Conventional desensitising therapy, based as it is on increasing massive doses of allergen (see page 96), will also cause EPD to fail and the two must not be attempted together.

Dr McEwen suggests a varying desensitisation schedule for different conditions:

1. Seasonal allergens (hay-fever etc), one dose per year, not more than four months before the onset of the season. If symptoms have commenced treatment can be undertaken but is less successful, unlike Miller's provocation-neutralisation method.
2. Dust allergies, two doses at an interval of two to three months.
3. Food and other allergies, doses at one, two and then three months (four times over six months); then boosters at four-month intervals.

Boosters may be used with any regime, where indicated.

Side-effects are remarkably mild, including redness and swelling of the arm, infections (at the site), pigmentation and scarring (at the site) and occasionally general debility. Rarely the person may feel profoundly ill for many weeks but even this effect wears off in time and happily does not denote a failure of the treatment (often the reverse).

By and large, conventional allergies, such as eczema, asthma, urticaria, migraine, irritable bowel syndrome and others, respond well. So far treatment does not seem to work for sensitivities to chemicals, drugs, food additives and stinging insects.

ALSO RANS

Some tests are mentioned here because you may encounter them. Nevertheless, they can be relegated to the category of interesting but not much use. The first two of these are considered scientifically sound by the conventional immunology camp. That is to say the results can be explained and fit in with accepted notions on the causation of allergies.

However, this does not mean that these tests are automatically of any intrinsic use. They rarely are. The RAST test, for example, is expensive and misses 98 per cent of useful intolerances. It is typical of the elaborate laboratory approach by hospital clinicians which clinical ecologists would consider no more than playing at allergies, an indulgence that can only be afforded by milking the health service financially and is simply another abuse leading to wastage of funds. The value of a test ought to be whether or not it leads to a recovery *not* whether or not it is scientifically supportable.

Radioallergosorbent (RAST) test

In this test, a known antigen, in the form of an insoluble polymer-antigen conjugate (usually a small impregnated disc), is mixed with the patient's serum. Adding radio-active iodine (I-125) labelled *anti*-IgE antibody and measuring the radioactivity taken up by the conjugate then gives a measure of the quantity of IgE originally present in the patient's serum.

Only Type 1 reactions (see Chapter 2) have circulating IgE, so that limits the test for a start. In some patients the test is dramatically positive to certain foods and other substances. There is no doubt at all that avoiding such foods will benefit the patient. The problem is that the test is often negative where there is a real demonstrable allergy and therefore the test is misleading.

Prausnitz–Kustner (PK) reaction

Sometimes it may not be possible to skin test a patient due to generalised dermatitis, extreme dermographism (skin wheals severely merely by being touched) or anxiety. In this situation it may be possible to use a surrogate individual. Antibodies are transferred by direct injection of the patient's serum from one individual to another and the second person then undergoes the skin tests. The results are equally valid.

Naturally, since blood is being injected from one person to another, it is important to screen for diseases such as syphilis, hepatitis and AIDS in the donor. Several 0.1millilitre amounts are transferred to different sites in a non-allergic subject (usually a relative). After forty-eight hours the surrogate may then be tested. (This means conventional skin testing and would not apply to the Miller method.)

Ophthalmic challenge testing

If the allergen being tested is one which affects the eye, it may be possible to perform tests by placing the suspect antigen directly on the conjunctiva. Apart from this consideration, it has no advantage over skin testing and is rarely positive when the skin prick test is negative.

A small amount of antigen (e.g. pollen in an aqueous extract) is applied to the lower conjunctival sac. A control is placed in the other eye, usually the diluent or some known unreacting substance. A positive response is characterised by burning, smarting, itching, oedema, or redness of the conjunctiva exceeding that of the control eye. If a positive reaction is obtained, the eye is irrigated with isotonic saline, then a drop of 1:1,000 adrenalin instilled.

It is quick but usually unpleasant for the patient, unless serial dilutions are used to follow, as per the Miller method. In this case the neutralising dose will stall any further unpleasant symptoms.

7

Acupuncture-related Techniques

THOSE CHINESE AGAIN!

Whatever discoveries are made in medicine, there is a strong chance that the Chinese thought of it long ago and have been using it successfully for centuries. I have already referred in Chapter 4 to the 'Chinese diet method' brought to my attention by my Japanese friend Dr Yukio Kitajima. Without actually using the term rotation diet or food allergy, it shows a clear-cut understanding of these two very important fundamentals of health.

Acupuncture is an ancient Chinese art that has gained much recognition in recent years. A number of medical practitioners have been to study it in the Far East and have become quite competent at it though, as with ink paintings, Kung Fu and stir fry, one is left with the nagging feeling that in some way the Chinese will always be better at it than we are.

It uses the natural wisdom of the body, indeed relies on it, to aid recovery and as such it may ultimately prove superior to Western scientific medicine which, except in a few useful emergency measures, seeks to overthrow the body's healing powers with potent drugs which incapacitate it or interventions which themselves cause permanent damage or loss to the body.

I do not practise acupuncture, nor do I propose to discuss its precepts here. There are now numerous texts for those who wish to know more about it and the reader is referred to these.

It is possible to be cured of an affliction caused by the allergic process, using acupuncture, without ever knowing what the allergy was. I am thinking of the fact that, for example, many arthritis sufferers experience a great remission in their illness after a course of acupuncture. However I am fairly certain that this approach will not diminish the allergy, merely mitigate the disease resulting. The allergic substance will continue to remain inimical to the body and retain its potential for future illness. But it does seem that, by fortifying the body's defences, an allergy is rendered less harmful. Referring to the content of Chapter 2 once more, it does appear that on occasion classical acupuncture may turn a stage 3 *maladapted* food or chemical into a stage 2, *adapted* one. Naturally, this is only an opinion and a great deal of work needs to be done to carry it from the realms of speculation into the real world of scientific fact (supposing that that could ever be achieved with something as mystical and close to the properties of raw Life Force as acupuncture).

What I want to discuss here is not acupuncture as practised in this familiar guise but two special developments of it which directly intervene in the allergy *diagnostic* approach; that is, these are means of detecting allergies, not of curing the disease process. Avoiding the allergen is still therefore the mainstay of the 'cure'. The first of these off-shoots comes from France, the second from the USA. It is exciting to think that unions of East–West knowledge such as these may bring yet newer aspects to both. I like to think that the deep intuitive wisdom of the orient is complimented by our radical enquiring attitude and that neither is superior, as it is sometimes fashionable to think.

THE AURICULO-CARDIAC REFLEX METHOD

One of the many interesting spin-offs from acupuncture to come to The West is this unusual approach to detecting allergies. I do not propose to go into the theories behind acupuncture – the body harmonies, energies and meridians, etc. – but to explain the technique purely in terms of known physiology.

Certain parts of the body have a cutaneous nerve supply which is innervated from the sympathetic nervous system and the rest of the body from its parasympathetic counterpart. Two sympathetic areas are the face in front of the jaw angle including the ear auricle, also the back of the hand. Nogier, an enquiring

French acupuncturist, showed that if a strong light is shone on these areas, a curious phenomenon is noticed when feeling the pulse; the site of maximum amplitude on the wave shifts downwards for several beats and then returns to normal. This is called a positive auriculo-cardiac reflex. Even more curiously, this takes place when something to which the subject is allergic is held near the body over one of the 'sympathetic areas'. Note it does not even have to touch the skin to produce this effect!

Thus the practitioner feels the pulse at the wrist and sites his thumb just beyond the tip of the wave travelling down the arterial wall. He then calibrates the reaction by shining a light on the back of the patient's hand, or on to the ear, so that he knows what to expect. In effect he feels nothing at first and then, as the pulse wave shifts, it comes down under his thumb and is clearly perceived. Normally there will be one or at the most four positive reactions.

All he then has to do is bring samples of foods one at a time close to the skin of, say, the forearm and note whether the pulse-wave moves or not. Note: *This has nothing to do with pulse rate, which rarely alters*. It is purely a change in the physical location of the maximum amplitude. Fig. 7 illustrates this.

Dr Julian Kenyon, of the Southampton School of Alternative Medicine, has refined and extended this technique with his associate George Lewith. They have produced a range of standard allergens, mostly food, in plastic test 'filters'. Since they have trained most of the British GPs who use this method these are what you are likely to encounter.

First a blank filter is used, in case the person reacts to the plastic itself. If this is the case then glass containers are used.

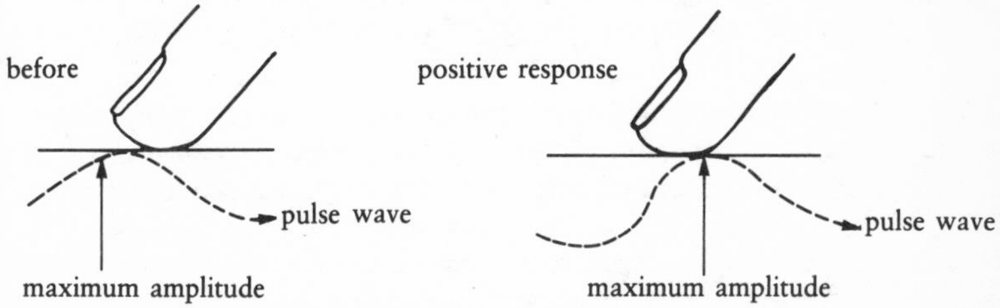

Fig. 7 *ACR method shift in maximum amplitude*

Then food and chemical samples are brought up, one at a time, and the response gauged. Kenyon and Lewith reckon that more than ten positive auriculo-cardiac reflexes indicates an allergenic substance and that thirty or over is a sign of a severe allergen. These are the only substances that they recommend the patient to avoid.

The advantage of this method is that it enables a large number of substances to be screened very rapidly, one a minute or even faster. This saves the practitioner's time and so, in economic terms, is less costly for the patient. Even if the method is not entirely accurate, and having experimented I believe provocation testing is certainly a shade more exact, it is certainly correct enough of the time to become probably the most cost-effective method of all. You don't need to locate 100 per cent of the patient's allergies to make him or her well; 75 per cent will do and the ACR method can certainly score that high, though it takes a degree of skill and practice which other methods do not require. This is a potential weakness.

It is difficult but certainly not impossible to carry out the ACR tests on children who may be fractious and un-cooperative when it comes to intradermal skin testing. This is clearly less disturbing for them. Also it may form a good preliminary to exclusion dieting in the young, the old or the severely debilitated patient, avoiding the rigours of the Stone-Age Diet or a fast. The patient only avoids those foods which cause a pulse effect.

It has been claimed that neutralising doses can be obtained using this method; progressively weaker serial dilutions are used until one is found which does *not* produce the pulse reaction. This is taken to be the neutralising dose. These drops may be effective, but several times I have tried injecting a sample per the Miller method and on occasion had a wheal growth and symptoms; not a manifestation that would be accepted for a neutralising dose on the Miller method (see Chapter 5).

Strangeness apart, this is a useful method. Clinical ecology doctors use it in certain centres and no-one doubts their commitment to its effectiveness. But I suspect it may be a long time before anyone can explain properly how it is mediated.

APPLIED KINESIOLOGY

While on the topic of acupuncture, we come to an even more peculiar and controversial technique, but one which is again easy to try empirically by anyone who cares to side-step their prejudices. It represents a bridge of a kind between oriental acupuncture theory and western chiropractice technique (osteopathy in Britain).

Chiropractice is locked in conflict with the medical profession in the USA, the bitterness of which is hard to understand here in the UK, where doctors have nothing to lose financially because of competition from alternatives. The fact is that physical manipulation is a safe (though not always gentle!) approach to health that can do little harm, may do some good and is not to be compared with the immense potential for damage that is the trouble with modern interventional medicine with its poorly understood drugs and readiness to cut and carve. The stories of chiropractors ruining people's health, circulated glibly by doctors from the USA whose very tone of voice often gives them away, seem a little far fetched to us this side of the Atlantic. Presumably there are bad chiropractors, just as there are incompetent doctors, but this is hardly reason to condemn the subject in such vituperate terms.

From the basic principles of chiropractice and acupuncture sprang another discipline called Applied Kinesiology (Greek: *kinetikos*, move), described and developed by George Goodheart, John Thie, David Walter and John Diamond. As its name suggests it is primarily concerned with the dynamics of posture and movement. In other words with muscle tone and performance. Although it has no proven scientific basis, it does seem to rest upon a certain body wisdom and, despite what was said about quackery earlier in this book, its techniques are beginning to interest a growing number of doctors (including myself). A simpler version for the layman, Touch for Health, was developed by California practitioner J. F. Thie and a contact address is given at the back of this book, if you want to find out more.

In brief, the Applied Kinesiologists showed that muscle tone is very variable and influenced by a variety of unsuspected excitants and depressors. The theory is that some of these muscles are related to the function of the acupuncture 'meridians' and reflect the general state or performance of that meridian. For example the psoas muscle is considered to be associated with the bladder meridian (not the bladder, but its meridian, note).

Almost all muscles have an opposite and competing muscle, the correct tension in each bringing about a balanced but dynamic state. In less than optimum conditions, this fundamental balance is lost and performance, posture etc. progressively impaired. AK has methods of restoring the balance in muscle performance, by selectively strengthening or weakening groups until the desired state is reached.

One remarkable finding is that allergenic substances held under the tongue, or even near or against the body, (compare this with the ACR method above) will cause a drop in power of certain muscles. This can be demonstrated with a high degree of consistency, even if performed double blind, that is with neither the practitioner nor the patient being aware of what is being tested. No one pretends to know the physiological basis of this effect, simply that it can be shown to exist.

Of course, given skill and practice, this provides a very useful and rapid method of screening for food and other allergies. The person is given a general 'balance', that is to say the body is brought as close as possible to optimum in overall muscle tone. This may only take a few minutes. Then one particular muscle or a group of muscles are selected and tested as a baseline tone. Dr Hugh Cox, a Berkshire general practitioner, suggests the following:

> Initially, six muscles are used in testing:
> 1. Clavicular head of pectoralis major.
> 2. Anterior deltoid.
> 3. Latissimus dorsi.
> 4. Quadriceps.
> 5. Psoas.
> 6. Tensor fascia lata.
>
> The technique is to test the ability of the patient to maintain the limb in a locked position when a firm pressure is applied for 2–3 seconds, testing all six muscles.
>
> Either arm or leg can be used.

Next substances are challenged one at a time by administering a sublingual drop and the muscles are tested again. Dr Cox says he began by using actual food under the tongue but was concerned that some patients might see or taste the food and those with an aversion to it might produce false positive results. Now he uses the Miller No. 1 solutions (i.e. 1 per cent). It only takes a matter of moments; after each test the mouth is rinsed out and the patient is then ready for another. Any foods which cause a sharp drop in muscle tone of any or all six muscles are assumed to be allergenic and the patient is told to avoid these. Non-food substances can be tested with equal facility.

An exciting idea is the use of surrogates in testing by this method. (Sceptics had better pass over this section!)

Basically a surrogate is used where the patient is either too young or too infirm to test reliably by the AK method. The surrogate is tested first, alone. This testing is then repeated with the surrogate holding the patient's hand, or in the case of a baby, it may be rested on the surrogate's body, if lying on a testing couch. Then the test solution is offered *to the surrogate*, not the patient. If the muscles weaken, this is accepted as evidence of allergy in the patient. This has nothing to do with allergies in the surrogate, whose own intolerances can be tested separately and are usually entirely different – if he or she shows any reactions at all.

Unfortunately, what the subject is thinking can influence the test. The surrogate therefore must concentrate somewhat on the patient. This is an unfortunate weakness of the method as a whole. If the patient thinks 'weak', this will influence the test. I have even heard it said that the practitioner himself can influence matters in this way. Thus carrying out the tests blind or double blind and repeating them several times may increase the accuracy.

The main point is that this is not offered as a highly accurate method but a rapid and useful one. In the National Health Service, where doctors are greatly overworked and funds are short, it has a great deal to offer. Dr Hugh Cox, himself a GP, is in a good position to comment on these advantages:

> Applied Kinesiology I believe is a useful tool in the investigation of food, chemical and inhaled intolerance for these reasons:
>
> 1. It does not require expensive laboratory equipment.
> 2. It does not require an elimination diet prior to testing.
> 3. It is less costly to the physician and the patient.
> 4. It is not invasive.
> 5. It is repeatable.
> 6. It is rapid.
> 7. Blind and double-blind studies can be conducted easily.
>
> The only limiting factor is one of inducing fatigue in the group of muscles tested. For this reason it is probably wise to switch to the opposite limb after ten to fifteen items. (In actual fact, I have rarely found this to be a problem).

AK lends itself to the layman non-doctor approach. A number of untrained people are setting themselves up and offering to test around fifty items in half an hour. You should disregard exaggerated claims such as these and bear in mind the weakness of this method which means that cross-checking is mandatory, even if it does slow up the procedure somewhat. In any case my overall advice in this book applies: that recovering from your illness may involve much more than merely identifying allergies.

BIOMAGNETISM

Biomagnetism is a relatively new discipline, based on the work of Osamu Itoh of Japan and Terence Williams, an extraordinarily gifted 'healer' in England.

It acknowledges the general acupuncture principle of harnessing the body's own energy for healing, by means of eight extraordinary meridians. But instead of applying needles, small magnets with gold and aluminium inserts are used at certain selected acupuncture points, which 'open' each meridian in a similar way.

This may be combined with other touch and 'hands on' techniques, such as *T'sien T'sju* (a means of rebalancing body energy by contact).

It is ingrained with oriental jargon such as the subtle bodies in the aura (spiritual planes beyond the merely physical body), the *Chakras*, *Chi* energy, conception vessel and the like. There is a common occidental tendency to disparage such mystical knowledge without even being aware of its precepts.

I have no comment to make on it, other than a general anecdotal one, which is that I have observed several patients recover from their allergic diathesis.

Ultimately, we should be asking ourselves certain questions, such as: why is it that the body generates allergies? Can we not simply *get rid* of the allergies, without worrying what they are, by reharmonising the body's energies so that problems are simply sloughed off. Clearly, this would be a better overall approach.

8

Auto-immune Urine Therapy

An interesting and startling new idea that you may encounter in the treatment of allergies is the use of the patient's own urine as treatment. It has been claimed to be a source of competent antibodies of value to that patient. In fact it could be a unique therapeutic agent, since only that patient's urine could possibly contain the exact correct antibodies to his or her allergens.

How this could be true and what practical value such a curious and on first sight unsavoury method might have is worth considering in more detail.

At least one film actress has given it media coverage and her claim that it has helped her, reported in popular magazines, has gone some way to making it more acceptable to the public – though this cuts no ice, as always, with the medical profession. I suspect it will become used more and more in the future and may eventually establish itself as a creditable treatment. Certainly, it has strong theoretical points which make it attractive and these are discussed below.

Actually, when I say 'new' this is quite incorrect. Drinking one's own urine therapeutically is a very old idea and its beginnings are lost in antiquity. Naturally, it has been dismissed as folk-lore, unworthy of serious study, by our modern self-illuminated boffins. Yet it is a curiously persistent notion – a fact that itself bears some consideration.

Dr H. Newbold of New York became interested in it and carried out a survey of the literature. He came across no fewer than 130 references to treatment with urine, the earliest scientific report dating back to 1863, *The Physiological Memoirs of Surgeon-General Hammond, US Army.*[1] But the paper which seems to have generated interest among a few fellow doctors was an account in 1947 by Dr Jonas Plesch, who was incidentally personal physician to Albert Einstein. He left Germany at the time of the Nazi takeover and set up a fashionable practice in London's Mayfair. Dr Carl Eckhardt of Riverside, California read his paper while on service in Europe during the Second World War and put it to the test when he returned home after demobbing.

He tried it out first on a member of his family with severe incapacitating eczema and it cleared up completely. From that time until his death in 1976 he carried out approximately 70,000 treatments of 9,000 cases with remarkable success and relatively few side-effects.

Today's leading exponent is probably Dr William Fife, from Sacramento. Fife himself was a sufferer and had been forced to retire due to ill-health. By chance he heard of AIU and after a course of treatment his health and vigour were restored. He resumed practise and now employs the method with many of his patients.

He claims that several clinical trials have shown that over eighty per cent of patients have experienced various degrees of clinical improvements, lasting up to many years without further treatment. However he does caution that it is wrong to talk of a cure. AIU lowers the individual's sensitivity and allows more contact with previous offending allergens but sensitivity is only reduced, not abolished, so frequent injudicious antigen exposure will still cause trouble. Thus the new patient expecting an immediate cure without regard to exposure and continuing their addictions will usually be disappointed. But the severely ill patient who has learned to be prudent will be grateful for this marked relief.

FIFE'S TECHNIQUE

The patient is given a sterile plastic urine container and a medicated swab with instructions on how to collect a sterile specimen of mid-stream urine. This is tested before use in the normal way for specific gravity, pH, glucose, proteins etc.

Ten millilitres of urine is then transferred to a syringe fitted with a micropore bacterial filter and the requisite amount of urine collected after filtration. The amount depends on the patient's build. Fife gives the following dosages:

TABLE 8.1 WEIGHT-RELATED DOSAGES IN AUTO-IMMUNE URINE

Patient's weight		*Dose*
over 90 kg	200 lb	8 ml
over 72 kg	160 lb	7 ml
over 52 kg	115 lb	6 ml
over 31 kg	70 lb	5 ml
over 18 kg	40 lb	3 ml
infant		2 ml

The patient is then placed face-down on the couch and the upper outer quadrant of the buttock cleaned with a swab. The needle is placed at a slant into the subcutaneous fat and the injection given very slowly over three to four minutes. Some patients find it less painful if two millilitres of 2 per cent Carbocaine (or Lignocaine in the UK) are added to the injection solution. The disadvantage is that this itself may be an allergenic chemical.

If the specific gravity is below 1.010, one to two millilitres extra solution are injected, except in infants. If the specific gravity is below 1.005 then the solution is probably too weak to be effective. Fife recommends that patients under intense emotional stress have the dose reduced by one third. In his view the correct dosage is critical to success.

Treatments are generally given once a week but it is not detrimental if one or more is omitted. The intervals need not be exactly one week, but usually this is convenient from the point of view of scheduling appointments.

Treatments are avoided during menstruation.

Observation shows that improvement is frequently manifest in two stages. One, almost immediate relief of symptoms, indicating an immune blocking effect; the other comes after several months, suggesting an antibody build up similar to immunisation.

ADVANTAGES

Fife lists a number of advantages for Auto-Immune Urine Therapy:

1. Extensive allergy testing for all possible antigens is not essential to treatment as the body makes its own antibodies to all the antigens it is reacting to. *The body does its own testing.*
2. A degree of self-perpetuation appears to be present. It acts like an immunizing vaccine. Optimum improvement occurs after several months.
3. The medication is cheap and being fresh no preservatives are required.
4. There are no toxic chemicals or drugs required for hypersensitive patients to have reactions to.
5. It is safe. A few minutes before the treatment the urine was a natural sterile constituent of the blood. Since it is autogenous, unaltered and the antigens have been attenuated by passage through the body the most sensitive patient is spared the danger of anaphylactic reaction. Over 100,000 treatments have been given in our clinics without a single serious reaction.

   Adverse reactions have been minor and limited to the flaring up of previously experienced allergic symptoms or the premonitory feeling of coming down with a cold, such as a slight headache, mild depression, and mental stimulation. This stimulation is appreciated by the tired and depressed but can be temporarily disturbing to some tense schizophrenics, so they should be under adequate supervision. These symptoms may last for a few days after a treatment.

   Rarely, a local inflammatory reaction at the site of the needle penetration occurs and may subside voluntarily or with the aid of an antibiotic injection. These are the only known adverse effects that have been encountered with our procedure. There is a notable lack of any local tissue destruction from the urine.
6. It is effective. Statistics in our own clinic show that 92.6% of the patients with the more severe easily observed allergic symptoms such as asthma, hayfever and eczema were relieved by 50% or more. The mean was 70% relief as reported by patients and our observations. The usual comments after therapy are, I feel stronger, I don't get tired and I can do more. I can eat more food without reactions. *The most severe allergies show the greatest response.*[2]

INCREASING THE CHANCES OF SUCCESS

Since the success of this treatment, theoretically at least, depends on the presence of effective antibodies in the urine, it is sensible to try to boost these just before treatment. Thus the patient is told to expose him/herself to moderate amounts of his/her known or likely antigens the evening before reporting to the clinic. This may mean eating several suspect foods or spending some time inhaling the air in suspicious locations. Foods expected to produce a severe reaction are not eaten until arrival at the clinic (the AIU injection will then probably switch off the symptoms quickly).

All fluids are avoided for four to six hours beforehand, to avoid diluting the urine.

The best time of all to collect urine is when the patient is at the height of a symptom attack. It may not be possible to identify any known or possible allergens for the patient but if, at the time of collecting the sample, the patient is reacting then it seems logical that at that time the urine will be loaded with antibodies. The patient may thus be told to report at once to the clinic if a reaction starts up.

As mentioned previously, there is little hope of success if the patient doesn't also carry out at least some corrective procedures in their environment and diet. Thus it is necessary to advise the patient to avoid addictions, such as drugs, tobacco, alcohol, coffee, cola, wheat, sugar, milk, junk food etc., as appropriate. Chemical fumes must also be avoided and dust or mould may need to be radically reduced in the home, depending on the nature of the problem.

For those not ill enough to give up their addictions (yet!), the diet should provide adequate fibre from whole grains, raw fruit, vegetables, nuts and seeds. A rotation diet may help.

AN ILLUSTRATIVE CASE

Dr A. P. Dunne of Ireland became a champion of the technique when she tried it on herself and found it worked. She makes a good model to recount the usual sequence of events in treatment.

> My personal experience with AIU was as follows. For many years I had multiple allergies, the number of which kept increasing. Wheat, beans and chicken caused depression, beef – paranoia, pigmeat – facial oedema with watering eyes and nose, dairy products – water retention, aerosols or cleaning agents – headache and wheezing, gas fumes – aggression and irritability and perfumes –

faintness. Solar dermatitis developed annually, contact with metals produced itchy eczema – I could not wear a watch, necklace or even my wedding ring – and bites or stings resulted in oedamatous weeping ulcers lasting for weeks. City air pollution produced such mental confusion that for seven years all my messages [groceries, etc.] had to be purchased in outlying shopping areas. Chronic symptoms became acutely disabling when exposed to emotional stress, and fatigue limited function to immediate priorities.

Following my return from the USA, I injected myself subcutaneously once weekly in the thigh with 4ccs of urine, using the Swinnex filter as described above for 4 weeks without, however, risking exposure to known antigens beforehand, as there was no allergist to monitor events. Four hours after the second injection, I experienced severe depression which tapered off without palliative measures in 2 days. After the fourth and last injection, I regained a degree of health that had been absent since the birth of my first child 25 years earlier. Though still careful with diet, I now eat moderate portions of formerly allergenic foods with impunity. Sunshine, metal or insects produce no reaction – and I travel in cities with a clear head. The real bonus was in cerebral function. New clarity of vision made me realize how blurred the old world had been. My deafness, which an Ear, Nose and Throat specialist had charted on his machine and which failed to improve with three different hearing aids, disappeared. Actions became spontaneous instead of the product of laboured planning. Memory, concentration, and decision-making had been so subtly impaired over a long period of time that only when these faculties became normal could I realize the extent of their erosion. Being unable to depend on one's mental function is the ultimate insecurity; after a quarter of a century of foggy existence I entered a clear world. One immediate objective change was in handwriting. My wandering scrawl, which had at times been so indecipherable that the bank questioned signatures, became regular, neat and clear.

In the 8 months since AIU self-administration no boosters were necessary as no deterioration occurred, despite wider exposure to allergens.[3]

The severe depression is worth commenting on. Fife doesn't mention it but it seems to be a frequent occurrence. Newbold remarks on it also.

Nancy Dunne is an accomplished writer, supplementing her income with frequently published entertaining fiction. Perhaps this skill is one of the reasons her essays regularly win prizes in the Action Against Allergy sponsored essay competition held annually and open to doctors. The above extract is from such a prize-winning essay. Having on a number of occasions dined with her in Dublin and listened to her never-ending store of enlightening medical cases, I consider her one of medicine's great story-tellers; though in part that could be due to the Irish national character of which she is a truly colourful and eccentric example.

THE ORAL APPROACH

As I have already commented, belief in the beneficial effects of drinking urine is lost in the mists of time, though for centuries this has been dismissed as a meaningless folk superstition, on a par with 'wing of bat and liver of toad' recipes. It is surprising therefore that modern science has shown that there is something to the myth after all!

Dr Dunne is worth quoting again on a modification of the method she tried which rather harks back to this ancient lore. Isolated cases do not make a scientific study. But they should, and often do, alert the enquiring mind to the possibilities.

> Shortly after my own experience, I modified the technique to treat a 5-year-old hyperactive male. Conor's itchy eczema which covered the entire skin surface was present from birth. His face and scalp exuded yellow fluid, his eyelids drooped permanently and his nails blackened and fell off. Patches of secondary infection from scratching produced frequent bouts of fever and local adenitis. He could not use his hands which were semi-closed crusted claws and his whole appearance was revolting. When kept in one position for any length of time he stiffened and was unable to walk. He had constant earaches and fits of hysteria, often damaging himself with head banging, and never slept more than half an hour consecutively at night. Specialists, hospitalizations and even forms of alternative medicine failed to give any relief. He was on regular antihistamines and sedatives and had many courses of antibiotics.
>
> I advised his mother to collect his midstream urine at the height of exacerbation of symptoms and, using an eyedropper, to place three drops of his urine under his tongue four times daily, propping his mouth wide open to prevent swallowing. The first time she used it he was having a screaming fit which normally lasted half an hour – within one minute this subsided and he relaxed totally. By the fourth day, there was noticeable discharge of viscous matter from the oedematous surface with the development of red spots everywhere. He also began each day with sneezing and coughing with flowing

> mucus. His mother became alarmed at the copius discharge but she was persuaded to persist, while at the same time tapering off Conor's medication. By the sixth day the red spots changed to white, clear patches of skin were appearing, his eyelids no longer drooped and he was sleeping 4 hours at a stretch.
>
> After 2 weeks, he was off all medication, able to use his hands and walk freely, and no longer developed asthmatic attacks near grass or neighbours' pets. I increased his drops to six *q.i.d.* [given four times a day] and he began to pass a much greater volume of urine daily with heavy whitish sediment. His hair darkened, healthy nails began developing and adults in his environment remarked how placid he had become with his peers. When he and his family emigrated two months later, his hyperactivity, hysteria etc. were gone – he was sleeping soundly at night for the first time since birth – and apart from two small dry areas behind the knees, his skin was completely clear and he was asymptomatic.[4]

It might be advisable not to tell the child if you are using urine as a therapy. Their discretion is proverbially bad and any misunderstandings can be avoided this way. Thus many people collect night and morning samples of urine and add a few drops to the child's food or drink, which is quite satisfactory.

According to the latest reports from Dr Fife and others now using the sublingual modification, improvement is much more rapid using a one in five homeopathic-type dilution. One drop of urine is shaken with five millilitres of sterile water, one drop of the mixture is added to another five millilitres and shaken and this is repeated three more times (five dilutions in all). The final dilution is made with 80 to 90 per cent proof vodka!

Three drops are placed under the tongue hourly until there is obvious improvement or exacerbation of symptoms. As improvement progresses the interval is lengthened between treatments. After three days, treatment is suspended, to avoid pushing the immune system too fast initially. The urine therapy stimulates the immune system and it is the recovery of resistance that ultimately restores normality, over a period. Treatment is resumed if progress remains static or relapse occurs.

DISCUSSION

Schmidt in 1954 passively administered certain antibodies to rabbits and found that this suppressed the formation of IgE (immunoglobulin).[5]

Matsumuro in 1970 began treatment of asthma with processed serum containing blocking antibodies mixed with known allergen, by repeated immunisation injections. He found that the patient blocking antibody titres increased significantly and that the patients improved clinically and remained symptom-free for an indefinite period of time.[6]

Many investigators have independently and unequivocally demonstrated the presence of physiologically significant functional quantities of competent antibodies in normal human urine.

Professor C. H. Wilson, of Dublin (now practising in Lanark), on hearing of William Fife's work, injected guinea pigs with their own urine and found it prevented anaphylactic shock when the animals were later challenged with allergens (the guinea pig is chosen for these studies since it is curiously susceptible to anaphylaxis).

Opponents of AIU say it may be dangerous and cite the findings of Lerner that acute glomerulonephritis can be produced in rabbits by injecting them with their own urine.[7] Fife points out that this happened only when the urine was altered chemically and concentrated. He adds that Lerner was unable to produce any disease by injecting normal, unaltered urine or even when one ureter was severed and opened into the perineum. Contrary to these fears, Purcell[8] reported the use of urine to have very therapeutic effects in the treatment of glomerulonephritis in children.

Probably one of the main reasons that urine therapy is not more popular than it is is the aesthetic objection in our culture. Also, like clinical ecology and holistic medicine in general, it suffers from lack of funds to research and develop it. While drug companies go on pouring billions into so-called research, much of which is nothing more than complicated advertising gimmickry, such safe and potentially beneficial methods as those in this volume have to get by on word-of-mouth and personal experiment by individuals with limited resources. One can only press on or, in my case, write books which disseminate available knowledge as rapidly as possible.

Will urine therapy establish itself? Only time will tell.

9

Hair Analysis as a Tool

It might seem strange including a chapter on hair analysis for trace elements in a book which is reviewing allergy treatments but this is not actually so. To begin with, copper and zinc metabolism have been shown to be very important in the disposition to allergies. Also, allergies rarely exist without concomitant signs of malabsorption and even malnutrition in the patient, providing the physician knows what to look for. If those are not reason enough, it is probably true to say that clinical ecologists constitute the bulk of individuals who use this technique to help their patients, though that is not to say that all clinical ecologists employ it; many do not. I myself find it useful occasionally but only in conjunction with other clinical findings.

The use of hair as a biopsy specimen is still very controversial and undoubtedly too much is being claimed for it at the present time. Even the most skilled of physicians can only use it as a general guide. Nevertheless, there is much valuable information to be gleaned by those who know how to interpret the results, *providing* this is done in conjunction with a scrutiny of the patient *as a whole* and not just hair in isolation.

Examination of hair specimens is not new, though the first subjects were hardly studied for health reasons, being well and truly dead. In forensic medicine it has been known for some time that certain minerals may accumulate in the hair and nails and this can be useful evidence in a consideration of possible murder, for example, arsenic is easy to detect this way. A number of significant murder cases have hinged on this vital piece of evidence. Earlier this century, British archaeologists, in conjunction with forensic scientists, began to study mineral compositions present in the corpses of mummies, even though they have been dead for thousands of years.

Only in very recent years, largely due to pioneer work in the USA, has it been realised just how important certain elements are in attaining, or maintaining, optimum health. Often these are required in only the minutest quantities and yet are vital to the integrity of the organism as a whole. Hence the name *trace elements* in biology and medicine. The importance of these substances has been known for years in veterinary medicine, for example zinc deficiency can cause animals to miscarry or it can originate stillbirths. Thus farmers are very keen to understand the role of trace elements, and supplement them where needed for maximum health and performance in their animals. It is something of a sad state of affairs that even now, except in the case of a few enlightened doctors and allied workers, this is rarely done for our own species – Man.

CONTROVERSY

Undoubtedly one of the problems in gaining an understanding and hence acceptance of the way trace elements affect our health, has been the difficulty in obtaining any accurate estimation of their presence in a normal human being. It now seems likely that argon torch photospectrometric analysis of hair will provide this much-needed tool, though it is still too early to define its role precisely. There remains much confusion on the part of both the public and medical profession regarding its correct use and limitations.

On the one hand, the official position of the AMA (American Medical Association) is that expressed by Dr Paul Lazar, MD in 1974:

> hair analysis, along with other tests, is a useful tool. But present scientific knowledge does not support the use of mineral levels in the hair for broad, sophisticated, subtle diagnostic purposes and certainly hair analysis is not desirable for routine use.[1]

Cautious words and a sensible counter to some wildly exaggerated claims (largely in the advertising of disreputable laboratories) that hair analysis can diagnose diseases such as diabetes, heart disease, cancer and arthritis, years before they manifest themselves clinically.

On the other hand, a number of reputable workers have extended our knowledge about the role of these trace elements and also verified the usefulness of examining hair in order to gain a knowledge of the total body burden of these vital substances. Ten years on, it is right to say the conservative views held by Lazar and a large number of doctors are now somewhat out of date. Facts have begun to overtake opinions.

WHAT EXACTLY ARE WE MEASURING

The difficulty with interpreting hair analysis results is being sure exactly what we are measuring. One source of conflict in opinions is that hair biopsy results don't correlate very well with blood serum levels, which have been used for a considerably longer period to measure at least the elements present in large amounts (what might be called macro-minerals, as opposed to micro-minerals); substances such as potassium and calcium. Proponents of hair analysis are not deterred and argue, rightly, we have no justification for assuming that blood levels are an accurate guide to the total amounts of any substance in the body, let alone trace elements. Since the body tends to regulate carefully the levels in the blood it could be maintained at an artificially high level while in fact the body is very depleted. This is certainly true of a substance like calcium, for which the body would rob the bones and cause them to become soft and weakened, rather than allow blood levels to fall. Cardiac arrest would be the result if it did. So why should the same not be true for copper or selenium?

In any case, workers in this field are quick to point out that the picture given by the blood, which changes almost from hour to hour, could hardly be expected to reflect results in the hair, which represent changes over many *months*.

By and large, blood analysis measures *extra*-cellular levels. Hair analysis more closely monitors *intra*-cellular or tissue storage levels. These would logically be presumed to be more important to health, though this is no more than an assumption.

PROS AND CONS

One of the great advantages of hair as a biopsy material is that it is easy to collect, non-invasive and therefore painless. It keeps indefinitely under normal conditions without deterioration and its mineral content can be relatively easily measured. Only about a gram is needed, which most people can spare without any visible sign of loss. It isn't messy and thus there is no objection to sending it long distances through the post for analysis. This means that a few centralised laboratories can handle the tests and standardisation from lab to lab is not such a serious problem.

Over many years and vast numbers of cases, records have been kept on computer and thus it is possible to study patterns in large numbers of examples of given clinical conditions. As these record banks grow, the pictures which emerge become ever more clear and statistically sound. Thus, due to this ease of handling by a few well-organised laboratories, research is able to progress rapidly and we are learning more all the time.

Another outstanding advantage of the use of hair is that the substances being measured may be anything up to two hundred times more concentrated there than in the bloodstream. This makes relative measurements (see ratios below) much more accurate and minor variations less significant statistically.

Some obvious problems present themselves in the use of hair in this way. Would it not be probable that hair collects atmospheric pollution (few people wear hats these days)? Lead from petrol is bound to get on the hair of city dwellers; would this not be confused with lead actually present *in* the body, which arrived in the hair via the blood? The answer is a probable *yes*! Of course, the samples are washed carefully to minimise this problem and this has been shown to remove most exogenous elements, without disturbing the biologically bound substances,[2,3] but no-one knows for sure that substances arriving externally do not bind themselves on to the hair biologically in a way which makes removing it by washing difficult if not impossible. Vigorous washing of the sample, to try and remove these substances, may leach out quantities of the minerals that are truly present, again rendering measurements inaccurate.

Then there are chemical treatments of hair, usually for

cosmetic reasons. Selenium is believed to be a very important trace mineral (see below) and measuring it accurately is of vital concern. Yet it is the chief 'gimmick' ingredient of a number of shampoos, such as Selsun. Similarly hair darkening compounds such as 'Grecian 2000', may add spurious lead levels due to their utilisation of lead acetate. Bleaching and cold waving will also considerably alter the true picture of chemicals present in the hair.

Complicated? It certainly is. There is a great deal of work to be done before many doctors are satisfied with the tool. Nevertheless, it seems certain that hair mineral analysis will emerge as an important diagnostic tool for the practitioner, given time. In the meantime, the main problem is not the controversy which surrounds it, but the fact that the majority of doctors know little or nothing about nutrition and singularly fail in that approach to health. Perhaps educating them to the vital need for correct vitamin and mineral status should come first. By then the accuracy or usefulness of hair analysis may be beyond dispute!

SKILLED INTERPRETATION

Nutritional medicine is largely holistically oriented, that is it takes into account the patient *as a whole* and not severally by symptoms. For this reason skilled interpretation of hair analysis results is required, taking into account all available data, especially *other* parameters of health. Presumably the patient is sick, otherwise he would not have reported for care, and thus there will always be concurrent signs on which to base an opinion. Indeed, it would be folly of the highest order to try and diagnose and treat illness purely on the basis of a hair mineral analysis. This is the sort of quackery that causes scepticism in the medical profession.

However, for those who have taken the trouble to acquire the skill, certain patterns begin to emerge and these can be useful in guidance. Some doctors gain a certain aptitude at drawing conclusions about the individual's life-style and genetic background, though it is doubtful if the ability will ever supplant merely asking the patient the correct questions!

The real skill, of course, comes in helping the individual to feel better and regain optimum health. This is the ultimate test of that skill, indeed the point of it all. Wisely judged, the hair mineral analysis results can give invaluable guidance, though it would be wrong to state the case any stronger than that.

So it still remains to date a subject of hunch, intuition and some skill, which is not really a satisfactory basis for objective scientific practice. In my opinion, this position is unlikely to change until many more years of research have given us insight into the complex relationships of findings to variables such as diet, age, sex, environment and hormone status.

THE RESULTS

The range of elements tested and the accuracy to be expected from each varies somewhat from laboratory to laboratory. The Hair Analysis Standardization Board was founded in 1981, sponsored by the International Foundation for Health Research and now a branch of the American Holistic Medical Institute, in order to draw up guidelines to try to overcome this problem. The committee has five members who, though not all doctors, could fairly be described as experts in this field, under the chairmanship of Elmer Cranton, MD. None of the members has a professional or financial interest in any of the laboratories which carry out commercial testing of hair samples. They have sought to make recommendations covering such topics as sample collection, washing, analytical procedures, defining normal ranges and clinical significance of results.

The Board divides the elements that might be included in an analysis into three groups:

1. *Elements of proven clinical significance based on hair concentrations*:

   calcium
magnesium } possible deficiencies
zinc

cadmium nickel lead	possible toxicity
chromium copper	significant toxicity, also deficiencies possible

2. *Elements suggested to have possible clinical significance based on hair concentrations*:

sodium
potassium
selenium
antimony

3. *Elements with unknown clinical significance because of absence of data:*

phosphorus	iron
manganese	molybdenum
beryllium	cobalt
lithium	aluminium
vanadium	tin
strontium	iodine
fluorine	silicon
silver	

Note: the committee is not saying that these chemicals cannot be measured accurately or that the clinical importance of some of these elements is unknown – sodium, for example, is well documented – it is merely commenting that it is impossible at this time to be able to relate *hair concentrations* to any known clinical entity.

A typical screen would include sodium, potassium, magnesium, calcium, iron, zinc, phosphorus, copper and cobalt; then a number of less well-understood substances, but which seem to be vital, such as chromium, selenium, nickel and manganese; then finally some laboratories add extra elements, such as vanadium and molybdenum, knowledge of which is very scant but which it is hoped will eventually be found to fit into a pattern and correlate with certain as yet unknown disease processes – an admirable foresight.

Next will come a range of toxic substances, those which would not naturally be present and fulfil no known purpose but which, on the contrary, are definitely detrimental to health, such as lead, mercury, cadmium and aluminium. Arsenic is often included in this range but seems to be widely present and, up to a certain level, almost a 'normal' finding. Excess quantities are naturally poisonous.

Finally a number of useful ratios are also provided, the significance of each being constantly scrutinised and up-dated. Most important is the zinc-copper ratio, which is discussed below.

ELEMENTS INDIVIDUALLY CONSIDERED

Of the twenty or so elements normally screened in a hair analysis, *sodium*, *potassium*, *calcium*, *magnesium* and *iron* are present in large amounts and are not considered trace elements. Referral to any standard text of physiology will give a guide to their functions in the body.

Elevated *calcium* indicates increased excretion of the mineral via the hair. Blood levels are always rigorously maintained but excess calcium may be deposited in the soft tissues, a condition known as calcinosis. It is drawn from the bones which thus become deficient and weakened (osteo-porosis). Incorrect calcium levels would indicate defective hormonal control).

Magnesium may be raised secondarily to high calcium levels. Often there is a relative deficiency instead. Magnesium has been called Nature's tranquilliser and lack of it may lead to over-activity of the nervous system.

Potassium and *sodium* imbalances are indicative of endocrine dysfunction, especially adrenal stress.

Copper is necessary to the formation of healthy blood tissues. However, excess copper is toxic. Wilson's disease is a rare disorder characterised by high copper levels. The more usual reason would be excess intake due to leaching from the water supply pipes.

Chromium forms part of the glucose tolerance factor. Deficiencies of it seem to be associated with juvenile-type diabetes and hypoglycaemia.

Manganese is also connected with glucose metabolism. It is also important in the production of sex hormones, in bone growth and in the development and the utilisation of vitamins B, C, biotin and choline. Deficiency is almost entirely due to food processing.

Zinc has emerged as a vital element in many biological processes. Deficiencies are now becoming commoner, due to soil exhaustion, food processing, excess consumption of wheat and use of the pill. Symptoms caused by lack of zinc seem to include: stretch marks, irregular menses, prolonged wound healing, delayed growth and sexual development (dwarfism), joint pains, inadequate peripheral circulation and poor skin condition. A lack of it is also often found in rheumatoid arthritis, though no-one knows the significance of this. Coffee consumption and high copper levels aggravate zinc lack. White flecks in the nails are said to be due to zinc deficiency.

Ironically, a raised zinc level may denote a deficiency. The postulated mechanism is that, since zinc is vital for hair growth, a deficiency causes a slowing of hair growth and time to collect more zinc deposits, even though the element is in short supply.

Selenium deficiency may increase the risk of developing cancer and also loss of elasticity in tissues such as skin, which leads to premature aging in appearance.

Cobalt has only one known function and that is its occurrence in the molecule of vitamin B12. Lack of this vital vitamin leads to pernicious anaemia and peripheral nerve damage.

Other elements sometimes screened include *vanadium* and *molybdenum*. No known function can be ascribed to these but perhaps a trend or association will emerge eventually.

It is impossible to give more than sketchy information about these several elements. New information is emerging all the time. For more details readers should consult one of the many texts extant on this topic. Passwater and Cranton's book is highly recommended.[4]

In addition, each laboratory usually sends out a booklet, or precis of information, with each sample received, which will also provide further guidance.

MOST USEFUL AREAS

Those who use the method frequently generally agree that hair analysis is accurate and informative enough to be useful in three main areas. These will now be dicussed briefly:

1. *Identification of exposure to potentially toxic metals* such as lead, nickel, cadmium, mercury, arsenic and aluminium. It has been shown that we have several hundred times the amount of lead and over a thousand times the amount of mercury in our bodies that primitive man had. Some workers, such as Professor Bryce-Smith, are convinced that we are already, most of us, exposed to fully toxic amounts of lead.[5] This is especially true of children, many of whom have smaller body weights and yet the same ambient exposure (higher body concentrations). Routine screening consistently brings back results of lead levels higher than is required to affect mentation and in many cases much higher than could be regarded as safe.

High levels of *lead* and other toxic metals have been found to correlate with symptoms such as brain damage, loss of memory, impaired judgement, violent behaviour, slowed reaction time, depression, fatigue and hyperactivity. Naturally, one must be cautious of reading causation into this association; it is not yet proved but highly suspicious. Exposures to lead include tap water, canned foods, peeling paints, traffic fumes, street dirt and house dust.

Aluminium is also a toxic metal. Aluminium cooking pans, which have become all the rage, are the principal source of exposure to this metal.

For some unknown reason, *cadmium* levels in smokers are double what they are in the rest of the population.

Mercury comes from organo-mercurial insecticides, dental amalgams, tuna fish from contaminated waters (industrial effluent) and certain antiseptics, fabric softeners, floor waxes, cosmetics, adhesives and plastics. Thus it is quite a common substance and yet excess mercury levels are known to have dire consequences, causing irreversible brain and nervous tissue damage. The phrase 'mad as a hatter' originated from the days when felt for hats was cured using mercurial salts. Long term exposure resulted in twitching, spasms and outright dementia. Minamata disease is a modern and distressing equivalent, named from the Japanese coastal town where this pollution disease was first recognised.

Industrial exposures are also a cause of increased toxic metal levels but these tend, on the whole, to be well regulated by law.

The worst exposures undoubtedly come from our general environment. This is ironic, in view of the fuss made about chemicals at work.

2. *Malabsorption*: Conventional medical thinking only recognises severe degrees of malabsorption, that is defective utilisation of food passing through the bowel, so that proteins, vitamins, minerals, etc. are lost, despite being present in the diet. Coeliac disease, caused by an allergy to gluten, usually presents as frank malnutrition. The bowel is so damaged by the allergic reaction that it ceases to perform adequately. Yet with a characteristic aversion to common sense, the medical profession never considers that there can be minor degrees of malabsorption or that other food allergies might have similar effects.

In fact malabsorption is very common and probably affects about a third of the population, especially those over thirty-five years of age, when the stresses of life have begun to leave their mark. It is easily detectable on hair mineral screening by a flattening of all or most results. Ratios may be relatively undisturbed but the absolute values are low. The minerals are simply not being absorbed correctly and neither, by inference, are vitamins and their co-factors, also vital for health and longevity.

The condition originates from poor functioning of the exocrine digestive glands and their excretions (enzymes). Despite television commercial propaganda about excess acidity, inadequate or lacking secretion of stomach acid is the more usual problem present. It can be corrected by supplementation with betaine HCl and pancreatic enzyme extracts. In the meantime, extra vitamins and minerals will be required to rectify the lack.

3. *The ratios*: Although the actual values found by hair analysis may be of debatable accuracy, ratios, that is the relative proportion of one element to another, are much more reliable. Even though there may be differences in technique from one laboratory to another, this would not affect a ratio.

Again, knowledge is still in its infancy but it does appear that certain ratios may give valuable guidance to the performance of certain aspects of physiology. For example the ratio of calcium and phosphorus provides important pointers to bone deterioration through osteo-porosis. Sodium and potassium disorders indicate malfunctioning of the adrenal gland, so-called 'adrenal stress syndrome' found in allergic conditions and hypoglycaemia.

But undoubtedly the most important discovery is the vital link between zinc and copper and the apparent consequences of a disproportion between the two. A high copper level may cause a relative deficiency in zinc, leading to any of the symptoms quoted above. Conversely, if zinc supplementation is too vigorous or prolonged, there may be an apparent lack of copper, leading to deficient blood production and possible impaired liver performance. This is thought to increase the potential for arteriosclerosis. Thus through pathways not as yet understood, these two elements are strongly linked in metabolism.

This is borne out by the increased frequency of (proportionately) high copper – low zinc in a number of diverse conditions, such as schizophrenia, criminal and violent behaviour, allergic diathesis and eczema.

Studies among psychopathic killers and other violent individuals in American penitentiaries have shown a significantly high incidence of zinc-copper abnormality.[6] This is certainly not the only dietary manifestation to result in such extreme anti-social behaviour – food allergy and hypoglycaemia are known to do the same thing in susceptible individuals – but this is an important finding which all those interested in social ills, as well as the medical ones, would do well to heed.

Supplementation of zinc assumes great importance in these and similar cases. Concurrent administration of vitamin B6 seems to enhance the desired effect.

CORRECTING ABNORMALITIES

Clearly, discovering abnormalities on hair analysis would be of little use if there were no way to correct what was found. Fortunately, this is often simply a matter of supplementation, where deficiences exist. However it is advisable to continue for a considerable period, perhaps twelve months or so. Deficiencies are slow to arise and cumulative. It is reasonable that correction will take similar long periods, especially in view of the likely malabsorption.

Exact amounts depend on age, sex, general health and other factors, not merely the supposed absolute measurement of a substance in the hair. This usually requires clinical judgement and is best left to the trained practitioner.

Toxic metals, if only moderately raised, may be removed safely though slowly by administration of simple chelating agents such as pectin (apple) and sodium alginate (seaweed). One to two grammes of kelp a day may be sufficient. If the problems seem more urgent or extreme, chelation with clinical drugs such as EDTA may be called for. This is a highly toxic substance and would only be used under intense medical surveillance. Usually it would not be resorted to without evidence of high serum levels, to support the excess levels in the hair.

In the same way that deficiencies can cause problems, so can too much of certain minerals and so supplementation must be carried out intelligently with this in mind. For example, as mentioned above, too much zinc will cause a *relative* copper shortage and may lead to anaemia.

Since this is a rapidly advancing discipline there is no point in quoting absolute standards which would probably be obsolete before publication, but for extensive particulars you are referred to Table 9.1.

Equally, it would be pointless to outline quantities for supplementation, which in any case depends very much on the individual case. But as a guide a suggested formula from the same book is quoted in Appendix 1. If you are working out supplements for yourself, you might find it useful.

TABLE 9.1 HAIR ANALYSIS INTERPRETATION

Element	*If this element is low your next step should be:*	*If this element is high your next step should be:*
Calcium	1 Check for low dietary calcium intake. 2 Check for excess phosphorus intake from meats, food additives, soft drinks or other sources. 3. Eliminate sources of trans-fat (hydrogenated) in diet.	1 Rule out recent hair bleach or permanent wave as cause of erroneous elevation. 2 Determine if excessive, prolonged calcium supplementation has occurred. 3 Determine if excessive vitamin D is ingested regularly.

HAIR ANALYSIS INTERPRETATION (*Cont.*)

Element	*If this element is low your next step should be:*	*If this element is high your next step should be:*
	4 Determine if vitamin D intake is adequate. 5 Assess whether gastric hydrochloric acid levels adequate. 6 Determine if any medications (antacids, laxatives, diuretics) are routinely taken which might impede absorption.	4 Evaluate dietary calcium/phosphorus ratio for possible relative calcium deficiency. 5 Reduce any excess phosphorus intake (meats, soft drinks, food additives). 6 Evaluate if protein intake is excessive. 7 Assess magnesium intake for adequacy.
Magnesium	1 Check for low dietary magnesium intake. 2 Check for excess dietary calcium or phosphorus intake. 3 Determine if any medication (antacids, laxatives, diuretics) or excess alcohol is taken which might impede magnesium utilization.	1 Rule out recent hair bleach or permanent wave as cause of erroneous elevation. 2 Evaluate adequacy of magnesium intake. 3 Determine if calcium/phosphorus ratio in diet is in proper balance. 4 Evaluate adequacy of vitamin B6 ingestion.
Zinc	1 Evaluate adequacy of dietary zinc. 2 Assess adequacy of vitamin B6 ingestion. 3 Assess adequacy of vitamin A ingestion. 4 Check for antagonism from excess lead, cadmium or copper exposure.	1 Rule out use of zinc-containing antidandruff shampoos as hair contaminant. 2 Check for extremely low dietary zinc intake. 3 Assess adequacy of vitamin B6 and vitamin A intakes. 4 Check for prolonged, excess zinc supplementation.

HAIR ANALYSIS INTERPRETATION (*Cont.*)

Element	*If this element is low your next step should be:*	*If this element is high your next step should be:*
		5 Possibly measure serum or urine zinc.
Copper	1 Assess adequacy of dietary copper. 2 Investigate possible excess zinc or manganese supplementation.	1 Rule out hair contamination from swimming pool use. 2 Rule out recent use of hair treatment or permanent wave as contaminant. 3 Investigate dietary copper exposure sources: drinking water, supplements, soft water from copper pipes. 4 Perform 24-hour urine copper determination, serum copper, ceruloplasmin (copper-binding protein). 5 May check other family members for heredity or environmental cause.
Chromium	1 Assess adequacy of dietary chromium, and assess if foods high in refined carbohydrate are depleting chromium stores. 2 Reduce excess refined carbohydrate intake.	1 Investigate occupational or other exposure source. 2 Evaluate 24-hour urine chromium.
Nickel	(Clinical significance of low nickel is unknown.)	1 Rule out hair contaminant from recent bleach or permanent. 2 Investigate possible environmental sources.

HAIR ANALYSIS INTERPRETATION (*Cont.*)

Element	*If this element is low your next step should be:*	*If this element is high your next step should be:*
		3 Consider 24-hour urine or blood nickel measurement.
Lead	The lower the better. Lead is a toxic element.	1 Identify and reduce sources of lead exposure. 2 If level is very high, rule out external contamination by checking pubic or axillary hair lead. Measure whole blood lead. 3 Can further assess exposure with provocative test using EDTA injection and measuring 24-hour urine excretion. 4 Ensure adequacy of protective essential nutrients; particularly vitamin C, calcium, zinc, selenium, chromium, manganese and fiber.
Mercury	The lower the better. Mercury is a toxic element.	1 Identify and reduce sources of mercury exposure. 2 If level is very high, rule out external contamination by checking pubic or axillary hair mercury. 3 Can further assess exposure using dimercaprol (BAL) injection and measuring 24-hour urine mercury excretion. 4 Ensure adequacy of protective essential nutrients in diet, particularly selenium.

HAIR ANALYSIS INTERPRETATION (*Cont.*)

Element	*If this element is low your next step should be:*	*If this element is high your next step should be:*
Cadmium	The lower the better. Cadmium is a toxic element.	1 Identify and reduce sources of cadmium exposure. 2 If level is very high, rule out contamination by checking pubic or axillary hair cadmium. 3 Further assess exposure with a provocative EDTA injection test measuring 24-hour urine excretion. 4 Ensure adequacy of protective essential nutrients, particularly zinc, vitamin C, iron and fiber.
Arsenic	(The clinical significance of low arsenic is unknown.)	1 Identify and reduce sources of arsenic exposure. 2 Recheck level in pubic hair to rule out external contamination. 3 Consider 24-hour urine test or provocative chelation test with dimercaprol (BAL), measuring 24 hour urinary arsenic output.
Sodium	1 Review dietary sodium intake for more appropriate assessment. Low hair sodium is not directly related to sodium intake.	1 Assess dietary sodium intake. Hair sodium does not correlate with sodium intake. 2 Determine if soft water high in sodium is consumed.

HAIR ANALYSIS INTERPRETATION (*Cont.*)

Element	*If this element is low your next step should be:*	*If this element is high your next step should be:*
		3 Consider possible hair contamination from heavy perspiration. 4 Determine if diuretic medication is taken. 5 Check for cystic fibrosis if clinically suspected.
Potassium	1 Evaluate dietary potassium intake and dietary sodium/potassium ratio for more appropriate information. Hair potassium does not correlate with dietary intake.	1 Assess dietary potassium level. 2 Determine if diuretic medication is taken.
Selenium	1 Ensure adequacy of dietary selenium intake.	1 Check for hair contamination from use of selenium-containing antidandruff shampoo. 2 Investigate for an occupational exposure.

SWEAT TESTING

It is probably true to say that it is far easier to interpret hair analysis results in conjunction with other corroborative tests, such as sweat analysis for mineral content. If this is combined with ordinary blood serum levels an even better grasp of the individual's mineral status is possible.

For example, take the anomalous behaviour of zinc. When

deficient it causes slowed hair growth and thus longer accumulation of minerals, which therefore may not appear deficient at all. Zinc may even appear abnormally high! By examining the sweat and serum, it may show clearly that zinc is low in one or more compartments of the body and this will readily show that the hair result is spurious.

Incidentally, it is sometimes claimed that slow hair growth can be detected by abnormally high toxic metals, which of course have time to accumulate in exactly the same way that metabolic minerals do. Dr Len McEwen and his associates have been able to disprove this notion. The mean hair lead levels in a group of patients studied were the same, whether there was a pronounced zinc deficiency or not.

The main drawback with sweat testing is that the patients must present themselves *in person* at the laboratory, unlike hair analysis. Since there are very few centres equipped to carry out this procedure, for the majority of patients this means considerable travel. It is possible that sweat testing will become more widely available in the future but until it does its use is confined to those living near a laboratory or for whom distance is not a deterrent.

HAIR DOWSING

The conclusion of this chapter seems an appropriate place in which to mention the use of hair samples for dowsing purposes. A number of agencies claim to be able to diagnose vitamin and mineral lacks *and food allergies* from a lock of hair sent by post. Usually this is done by dowsing, that is dangling a pendulum over the hair and interpreting its movements.

It is unfortunate that practitioners of this method don't make it clear how they obtain their results. Undoubtedly large numbers of people each year pay a fee and send off a sample, believing the service they are paying for to be a properly accredited 'scientific' method, similar to the spectroscopic analysis. Whether or not you accept the validity of dowsing or its accuracy depends on your belief in 'vibrations', ESP and similar phenomena. It would certainly be narrow-minded of me to dismiss such techniques out of hand when many of my colleagues are equally sceptical of clinical ecology, largely based on prejudice and ignorance of the facts. My only wish is to point out that there is a fundamental difference of approach. If you are not sure, ask if the service you are considering using is based upon dowsing. Certainly if, as is sometimes the case, it is undertaking to diagnose allergies also from the hair sample, you may be sure that it is.

10

Cleaning Up Your Environment

A gazetteer of hints

Few people recognise the extent to which our environment has become chemically contaminated in recent years. With rapid advances in science and technology since the last war we have been swept along on a tide of chemicals which have entered our water supply, air, food, home, places of work and recreation centres. In other words it is impossible to be free of them.

The trouble is that it has all taken place so quickly that there has been no time to assess the danger factors in most of these exposures and it seems that we are to find out the hard and bitter way what perils we have put our delicate bodies in. I'm not thinking of the major disasters, such as Seveso and Bhopal, but rather of the story of blights such as blue asbestos, thalidomide and 2,4-D. How many other chemicals are waiting to be revealed as damaging, but which in the meantime we are all exposed to, is a matter for conjecture, but considering the thousands of chemicals with which most of us are in daily contact the chances are there will be many. Too many.

Perhaps we should take warning from those people who already feel ill on contact with many of these chemicals. Dr Hamlyn of Ivybridge in Devon compared them to human canaries. Like the birds that were taken down the mines to give early warning of poisonous fumes, perhaps they are telling us, if only we would listen, that we are facing disaster. What for them is poisonous and unpleasant in small quantities, will surely be bad for us all. Don't forget the essential element of time: although you may not feel adverse reactions on a day-to-day basis, what about the effects over many years as the toxicity accumulates? It seems highly probable that the deleterious result for us then will be just as bad as it is now for those already affected. This cumulative effect is especially important for children. Firstly they have longer to live and so face greater exposures. Also they have smaller body weights and consequently the same exposure will produce a far greater concentration in their tissues. The toxicity is thus proportionately higher and the long term effects are likely to be more serious.

Government bodies and many so-called scientists are misleading with their reassurances – are they waiting until enough people have been hurt and permanently damaged before they will see any 'proof' that these substances are harmful?

I'm afraid that in the meantime, it is rather up to us as individuals to do the best we can to combat this tide of personal pollution. To that end I have prepared this chapter, just to give you some idea of what you are up against. It is by no means an exhaustive treatment. I could have written a hundred times as much and still not covered everything. For one thing, I have not discussed exposures at work, not because this isn't an important area of contact for allergics – indeed it is probably the worst – but because it is very difficult for the individual to effect changes. Instead I have concentrated on diet and the home environment where, to a certain extent, you are in control of chemicals and other unwanted exposures.

Specific advice is given with some of the entries but, by and large, the message is 'avoid it if you possibly can'. If you can't cut it down to a minimum.

AEROSOLS

The modern aerosol spray can is a fairly recent phenomenon, yet in a short space of time has become almost ubiquitous. We now have hair-sprays, deodorants, polishes, waxes, air-fresheners, paints, varnishes, glues, glitter, party streamers, starches, stain removers, insecticides, anti-fungals, anti-perspirants, fertilisers and scores of other items available for instant easy spray.

Unfortunately, despite the variety in ingredients, the propellants are all virtually the same and *highly allergenic*. The fluorinated hydrocarbons used are truly inimical chemicals and more and more people are realising that they are adversely affected. Some patients cannot even enter a room where a spray was used a week before without being subject to an immediate asthma attack or some similar reaction.

Effects vary enormously and can include the whole gamut of allergic reactions, but brain dysfunction, such as stupor or confusion, is quite common. It is deplorable therefore that these items are used liberally in schools, both as adjuncts to cleaning and for 'removing smells' (most leave a smell that is worse than ever, supposedly disguised with some floral or 'natural' fragrance). This abuse has disastrous consequences for many children, who thus cannot concentrate. They perform poorly and are often scolded, when the real trouble goes unsuspected.

If you have aerosols in your environment, if you qualify as an allergy sufferer per the criteria in chapter 3, remove them all forthwith. No amount of convenience can outweigh the threat they pose to your health.

It may not be simply a question of your own personal use of such sprays but what others do around you which will have a part to play. If your wife uses hair-spray or a member of your family uses spray-on deodorant, *get them to stop*. Until you realise the menace, you may be puzzled by strange reactions: for example, passengers in a car are often known to start up an allergy reaction due to hair spray worn by another traveller in the same vehicle.

There is a double catch which is that you may not only react to the aerosols themselves, but that these may also provoke reactions to other foods and chemicals. In other words, eating a food could cause a maladaptation reaction after exposure to an aerosol, though it would not have done so otherwise. Allergy testing and investigations could then fail if you are allowing these compromising chemicals into your environment.

ATMOSPHERIC POLLUTION

The air we breathe today, especially in cities, could hardly be awarded the term fresh air. It is so corrosive that it damages the fabric of our buildings. Stop a moment and think what it must be doing to animal life at the same time.

The fact is that if you are allergic, you are quite likely to suffer intolerance of these fumes as part of your general diathesis. Many patients experience a dramatic improvement in their tolerance of food and other items when they get away from city life. This may be true for you. Holidays abroad sometimes give the clue: if you can eat and drink widely without ill-effects when you are in, say Greece, or Spain, this may be the reason.

The comprehensive environmental unit (page 113) is the only way to diagnose definitively these problems, but until these are widely available there are one or two things you can do. Firstly, if you suspect atmospheric pollution and your diet is reasonably under control, go away for a few days in the country or, even better, abroad. If you improve markedly, you have pin-pointed something about your home environment.

The trouble may be within the home or outside of it. To establish which with a fair degree of certainty, on the day you return home stay *outside* your house for several hours. Walk around, expose yourself to traffic and other fumes. If you feel ill before going indoors, then clearly the problem is atmospheric pollution.

Four to twenty grammes daily of ascorbic acid (vitamin C), depending on tolerance, may enable you to combat the worst effects of atmospheric pollution. Miller's neutralising drops to synthetic alcohol I have also observed to be helpful.

Best of all, if you can manage it, is to move to a less polluted area. This might seem drastic, but most people who have done it reckon that it was preferable to a lifetime battle with ill-health.

BATH WATER

See the section on tapwater for hazards. A number of conditions are made worse by tap water and, of course, taking a bath comes under this. Eczemas often suffer an exacerbation of symptoms after bathing. One patient, after months of inconclusive treatment, finally admitted that he felt better after taking a bath. If you remember that allergy may well equal addiction as discussed earlier, there will be no prizes for guessing he was allergic to tapwater! He made a dramatic recovery on discontinuing this mode of hygiene.

Taking a shower is often a *worse* alternative, since you are spraying hot water loaded with chemical straight on to the skin. The only tip I have which usually helps is to draw the water as hot as possible, without adding any cold, wait until it cools to tepid and then take your bath. In the interval, chlorine and some other substances ex-gas and are present to a lesser extent in the water.

I have heard it reported that sodium thiosulphate (photographic hypo) in the water diminished the effect, which is logical as it combines with it chemically to remove chlorine, but I have been unimpressed by the results.

I can't bring myself, as Dr Cedric Wilson of Carluke does, to tell the patients not to bathe at all. He maintains that by so doing we avoid many noxious chemicals which themselves give rise to body odour and that this clears up. Please yourself.

The most I do is to say avoid bathing for a test period. At least if you feel better then you know what it is you are up against!

BREAD

Long known as the staff of life, bread is actually a food which causes a great deal of ill-health, due to the widespread prevalence of wheat allergy.

Ironically, many allergy patients can eat white bread whereas the brown or wholemeal variety may make them ill. In fact, this is not as paradoxical as it seems at first sight. Wholemeal flour, by definition, is pure wheat. White flour on the other hand is so refined that many of the characteristics of wheat are lost.

Thus if bread is hard to tolerate, try the white variety. But you are advised to get it from a small local baker who can guarantee that it does not contain preservatives and other unnecessary ingredients. 'Improvers' are a trick. They bulk up the bread and enable the baker to sell you a bigger loaf with fewer ingredients (for more money, of course). Just another ploy using redefinition of words, Orwell's *Nineteen Eighty Four* style. They are a health hazard and certainly do not improve bread for the allergic patient.

The best bread is that which goes stale and is uneatable next day, such as the French stick or baguette. That means it has no preservatives. Remember, what kills mould will certainly harm you. Once again, this is completely the opposite of the usual propaganda about a food item.

CAVITY WALL INSULATION

Urea-formaldehyde foam insulation (UFFI) is a cause of considerable health problems; so much so that it has been banned in the USA yet, typically, we are still being told it is safe here in the UK.

For many years it gives off formaldehyde fumes which will cause unpleasant reactions in sensitive individuals. Thus the official cant that it is 'harmless' is once again meaningless, because we are not talking about fatal amounts but those required to make a person ill. The reassurances do no good if you are among the unlucky ones to whom formaldehyde is a potent allergen.

The trouble is that a house is a considerable investment and cannot be altered or disposed of lightly. Certainly do *not* buy a house with UFFI if you have allergies. And if you have a chance to leave one which has, take it. It is not possible to remove it once present, therefore if you suspect it is making you ill but moving is out of the question, you have a problem. The final answer is that you *must* move if you value your health, no matter how unbearable this is.

In making up your mind, try to assess the time-coincident factor in the onset or worsening of your symptoms, as against your exposure to UFFI. If you only developed symptoms after (maybe up to two years after) moving to a house with UFFI or having it installed, get out.

See *The Food Allergy Plan*[1] or *Chemical Victims*[2] for more about formaldehyde.

Most other cavity wall treatments are just as bad for the allergic patients. Glass-fibre, for instance, is a disaster for some.

Fluffed mica seems to be the least offensive material from the ecological point of view.

CIGARETTE SMOKE

This is a potent allergen and may cause you baffling reactions unless you keep it in mind.

Mandell and Phillpott[3] found it caused psychotic reactions in a significant number of inmates (10 per cent) at the Fuller Memorial Sanitarium in South Attleboro, Massachusetts.

Freedom from this peril may not only include your own personal habits but those of your immediate family. It may be very difficult to get them to give up the habit when they are not the ones who are ill. In the meantime, crowded smoky bars etc. may be out of bounds, but for most this will hardly be deprivation. As time goes by legislation geared to making smokers the outcasts, rather than non-smokers should help.

CLEANING MATERIALS

Remember modern cleaners such as detergents are potential hazards. Some of them are extremely powerful and you are well advised to avoid them. There are always simpler alternatives, even if they do call for a little more manual effort. Sodium bicarbonate can often be made to serve where more powerful alkaline agents, such as caustic soda would be used. Kleeneze supply a washing powder without any odorisers. Avoid 'biologicals' like the plague. Simple soap flakes will create a lather as surely nowadays as they did fifty years ago!

For personal washing use Simple, Castille or Neutragena soaps.

For household duties try soft green soap (that's its name!) obtainable from chemists. Twice As Gentle is a brand to look out for also.

CLOTHING

Without being able to draw hard and fast rules, most people are better off in natural fabrics, such as wool and cotton. Man-made fabrics all give off fumes long after they are new, especially in conditions of warmth such as is likely with garments next to the body.

Of course some people are allergic to natural fabrics also and trial and error is required to find what suits you best.

Unfortunately, almost all new fabrics these days are treated with formaldehyde, either as a dye fastener, crease-proofer (permanent pressing) or moth repellant. If you tend to feel ill in textile and clothing shops this could be why. Try to get rid of as much of the dressing as possible by frequent washing before putting new clothes into service.

COOKING UTENSILS

Allergics should avoid using non-stick pans with Teflon-type coatings. Such fluorinated hydrocarbons pose serious problems, as mentioned under aerosols (see page 165).

Similarly aluminium cook-ware is not recommended. See the chapter on hair mineral analysis. Evidence is accumulating that mysterious symptoms of the allergic kind may trace to aluminium contamination of food. This may be difficult to detect, since it will cause false reactions to many foods.

Glass (Corning Ware) and enamel are much to be preferred.

CROP SPRAYS

Last year there were over 1,000 million gallons of pesticide spray dispensed on to farming land. According to Dr Jean Monro of Friends of the Earth, reporting for the Pesticide Action Network UK:

> It is now impossible to get away from pesticides, 97–99% of all our vegetables and cereals are sprayed with one or more pesticides. Vegetables receive as many as 46 applications in a season, yet residues are hardly monitored and there are no legal limits.
>
> Up to 64% of the pesticide applied to wheat may end up unaltered in your loaf of bread. Some chemicals banned or restricted in many countries around the world and widely accepted carcinogens in animal tests or other health hazards, are still widely cleared for use by the official Pesticide Safety Precaution Scheme.[4]

Actually, as Dr Jean Monro points out, the term pesticide is a misnomer, a con: there is no such thing as a selective poison. What will kill bugs and moulds will also kill you and me. The correct term is biocide, something which kills life. Using the proper terminology would probably make far more people uncomfortable about this mass decimation of our environment. Perhaps then there would be less lethargy among the powers that be to the scale of this blighting concern.

Dr John Laseter of New Orleans regularly carries out blood screening tests for microscopic traces of important toxic substances used as pesticides and routinely finds such toxic agents as 2,4-D, Dieldrin and Heptachlor. In fact he goes further and says it is rare today *not* to find these pollutants in significant measurable levels in the human body. Remember that for some people it can take very little of a chemical to make them profoundly ill.

What can we do? Actually very little. It is an enormous sociological/political problem with the might of vested interest and totally commerce-oriented governments on the one hand and the conscientious worried citizen on the other. I do not presume to hold the key to this conflict of interests. I am merely trying to state the extent of the problem as a doctor and give you some idea of what you are up against. There is nothing more dangerous than ignorance in this instance.

In the meantime the problem, from the allergist's point of view, can be simply stated – eat as much uncontaminated food as you can. Be aware that even so-called fresh food is also chemically contaminated and may be dangerous to your health. Washing the foods thoroughly may help but will only reduce the general burden and will not usually remove enough chemical to avoid an allergy reaction if you are sensitive. It is a question of learning what you can and trying your best to avoid excessive exposures.

DUST

Housedust – consisting mostly of fabric fluff, disintegrated organic matter (such as insect and bacterial bodies), moulds, food particles, human skin scales and pet danders (where present) – is a potent allergen and has been well-known as such for a long time.

House-dust mite is an even more virulent allergen, possibly the worst of all for human kind. Except over about 18,000 feet altitude, it accompanies us wherever we go, generally accumulating in bedding which is warm for many hours a day and also contains a great density of skin scales, on which it feeds. On occasion, however, its multiplication can be so extensive that it settles as a fine white dust in many parts of the house, like talc.

If you know, or suspect that you are allergic to dust, it is vital that you make an effort to eradicate it as far as possible. Do not simply rely on desensitisation or neutralising drops of the Miller type without tackling the problem of exposure.

However, as any housewife will tell you, total eradication of dust is impossible. It is logical therefore to concentrate one's efforts where this will do the most good. Since we spend approximately a third of our lives in bed, the bedroom thus becomes the natural target area. Remember this is also where the mite is predominantly found. Attack is based on cleaning procedures and reducing the number of sites in which dust can gather. The use of ionisers is also discussed briefly.

1. First begin by removing as much fabric and other dust-gathering objects as possible from the room. Depending on the severity of the problem, you may want to go the whole way as follows:

no carpets (linoleum or wooden floors – but be on guard for allergies to pinewood, linoleum fumes etc.);
no curtains – use blinds;
no pelmets;
no lampshades;
no open shelving with books etc. – use cupboards and storage boxes;
cotton or low-fluff linen;
duvet instead of blankets.

In older buildings cracks will need to be sealed and this may mean resurfacing the floor before any kind of finish is contemplated.

2. Cleaning should consist of frequent vacuum cleaning and damp dusting with an antistatic fluid but *not* from an aerosol. The cleaner should have a good seal at the bag, otherwise it will create as much dust as it removes. The tube attachment should be used and the beater action is definitely out.

Undoubtedly the best machine is the American 'Kirby'. Although expensive, it is a superb technical achievement and you should consider it seriously as an investment. A representative will usually gladly give you a demonstration which includes actually sucking skin scales and mites out of the mattress into a glass receptacle. The sight is quite impressive. If you can afford one, so much the better. If not, some clinics may be able to hire you one at a modest charge, for a monthly 'blitz' on the problem. (I have no financial interest in making this statement.)

3. Many claims are made for ionisers, one of which is that electrostatically charged particles are removed from the air in the room. Acceptance is variable; evidence inconclusive. This does not mean they are not worthwhile – it means simply that you will have to try one out for yourself to see if it brings any relief

from dust-related symptoms. That's the only way you will be convinced. Beware, however: it could make you *worse*.

4. *Miticides* There are one or two products on the market which kill mites (see pesticides above for reservations on that matter). Nevertheless, these are being marketed for asthmatics and you might care to try this approach. Several sprayings are needed to kill the mite and continued vacuuming to clear the residual droppings. Thus the beneficial effects do not begin for several weeks.

My advice is to use miticides only if you are sure that dust mite is a severe allergy problem and you are quite confident that chemicals have no detectable bad effect on you.

ELECTRO-MAGNETIC FIELDS

It is becoming increasingly obvious that a number of people are made ill in the presence of electro-magnetic fields. Recently alarm was spread when a doctor pointed out a high incidence of suicides which could be plotted along a narrow corridor across the countryside which followed the line of a high tension electricity cable. But there are many more instances of a less serious and dramatic nature.

Electro-magnetic activity around high tension cables is easy to demonstrate. If you carry an ordinary domestic fluorescent tube near one on a dark night you will be able to observe it glow over a hundred metres away. People, it seems, are far more sensitive and detect effects up to three times that distance.

Nor is it confined to high pressure voltages. The ordinary domestic supply can have deleterious effects for some unlucky individuals. This applies to cables within the home and also to electrical apparatus, such as televisions, cookers, dishwashers and the like. The effect is made worse if the subject is in a field between two appliances, such as would happen with equipment fitted at opposite sides of a kitchen and the individual stood between them.

Cables are best conduited and twist-wrapped wires are best, since the two fields within the core cancel each other out, but unfortunately this type of wiring no longer conforms to British Standards for cabling.

One moral is quite clear: do not reside within half a mile of overhead electricity cables.

Incidentally, all this is part of the allergic diathesis. If the environment is cleaned up and diet controlled, tolerance of electric fields rises proportionately, which is what we would expect when we are dealing with the *whole* person.

ENERGY EFFICIENT HOMES

One of the worst things to strike our human habitat is the advent of energy efficient insulation. It may be great on the purse but ruinous for health; we become isolated ecologically and subject ever more to our own indoor pollution.

In former years draughts kept us well protected from accumulations of obnoxious substances in the air. Now these are not being dispersed. Add to that the fact that there are today legion chemicals present in the home, given off from plastics, man-made fabrics, paints, heating systems (ducted air seems to be the worst), cosmetics, aerosols etc., on a scale never before encountered and you realise the severity of the problem.

Modern offices are amongst the worst imaginable environments to work in. Down a coal mine would be more comfortable than many. Clinical ecologists now recognise a 'sick building syndrome' caused by extensive indoor pollution made worse by sealing out natural fresh air and circulating 'treated' air, such as from air-conditioners. It can cause inexplicable but extremely unpleasant symptoms, including severe mental disturbance.

An architect once boasted he could design a home that would cause a couple a divorce, so beware! These are not trivial considerations. In the meantime, get plenty of fresh air; open all the doors and windows you can stand. Start a movement against energy saving and be prepared to move if your state of health warrants it.

Radiated heat is less likely to cause problems than convected or ducted air.

FLUES

Chimney flues may present problems. Often these leak and give off serious fumes (see Indoor Pollution, p. 178 and Atmospheric Pollution, p. 166). Unfortunately, due to house design, most flues run through the bedroom wall on their way to the roof and it is here that the most significant build-ups may take place.

Ancient mortar may crumble and break down until it leaks quite badly. There have been many tragedies over the years of seeping fumes reaching a level sufficient to kill families while they slept unsuspectingly. Remember that all toxins can be allergenic to those who are sensitive, even in tiny doses; so be warned.

Even a new building is suspect if you can establish (a) that you are indeed sensitive to fumes and (b) those rooms with a flue make you worse.

The only safe course is to have the flue lined with a modern metal flexible tube liner which, although expensive, can be passed up the chimney with the minimum disturbance and mess.

Better still change to electrical radiators and eliminate gas or open fires.

Or move.

FOOD ADDITIVES (see also Appendix 2)

It is possible to write a whole book about food additives. Indeed several people have; for example:

Why Additives? devised and edited by the British Nutrition Foundation (Forbes, London, 1977)

E for Additives, Maurice Hanssen (Thorson's, Wellingborough, 1984).

Clearly it is beyond the scope of this gazetteer to do more than mention them as a generalisation. The main advice is to avoid them if at all possible and, in the most sensitive cases, at all costs.

Possibly the most fatuous justification for food additives I ever heard was at an annual conference of the McCarrison Society in Scotland (Dundee, 1983). A representative of the food industry addressed us and tried to argue that food had *no* nutritive value if it did not get eaten and thus, if it weren't for the attractive colourings and packaging of foods, with preservatives to keep it fresh longer, manufactured food wouldn't be eaten at all and therefore all these additives were actually contributing to the nutritional value of the foods! What this foolish lady did not appreciate is that doctors like myself would be only too happy if the food did not get eaten. People wouldn't starve, as she seemed to intimate, but would simply eat fresh wholesome food instead!

The Ministry of Agriculture and Fisheries produce a booklet, *Look at the Label*, which explains about food labelling and lists the main 'E' number ingredients. It is available free of charge from:

The Ministry of Agriculture, Fisheries & Food,
Publications Unit
Lion House
Willowburn Trading Estate
Alnwick
Northumberland NE66 2PF

The Soil Association produces its own contentious and informative booklet, *Look AGAIN at the Label*, available from 86–88 Colston Street, Bristol, BS1 5BB.

GARAGES, INTEGRAL

Petrol fumes are a common concern I find. It is bad enough to have to go out on to the street and expose yourself to noxious exhaust emissions. It makes less than sense to bring the automobile into your home, which is what integral garages effectively do. Fumes inevitably leak into the house and cause major pollution.

It isn't really enough to keep the outer doors open. It is far better (if you are already stuck with an integral garage) to park the car outside and to use the garage to grow mushrooms or for a model workshop. It's safer!

HOUSEPLANTS

Indoor vegetation can be a problem. I am not thinking so much of allergies to the plants themselves, such as the well-known primula allergy, but of moulds.

The soil in plant pots is a natural feeding ground for moulds, which require warmth, moisture and organic matter and which are present there in abundance. See the section on moulds in general, but you will need to be aware that many conditions from mental confusion, to asthma and eczema may get better by abolishing house plants!

Lending them to neighbours for a trial period is rarely conclusive and you will have to work at eradication of moulds in general, especially if you have already been diagnosed as having a mould allergy by a clinical ecologist.

INDOOR POLLUTION (See also Energy Efficient Homes)

A good clue to the fact that you may be suffering from indoor air pollution is that you are worse in winter. Hay-fever sufferers, as you know, have their peak in the warm months. A number of allergy conditions have no seasonal element (for example perennial rhinitis). But those who get worse in winter generally do so because of the build up of indoor pollution at that time.

When the weather turns cold we retreat indoors and close all the windows and doors. Draughts are discouraged and often sealed against. Then we turn up the heating systems, such as gas fires and stoves, which themselves are the principal causes of the pollution. Naturally, other obnoxious substances in the home like formaldehyde (see Cavity Wall Insulation, page 169) and Dust (page 172) also increase in concentration. Some tests suggest that carbon monoxide levels in the home may rise by as much as 200 per cent at this time. Yet quite small amounts of this poison, breathed over a period, have serious effects.

The moral is quite clear. Get plenty of fresh air, even in the middle of winter. Open doors and windows as much as you (and those you live with) can stand. Don't huddle over stoves and fires. Change your heating system, if practicable, to less polluting types, like electrical oil-filled radiators.

See the section on atmospheric pollution (page 166) in general for advice on testing for this phenomenon.

IONISERS

See remarks under Dust (pages 172–4) above.

MOTOR CARS

We spend a great deal of our time travelling in vehicles propelled by the internal combustion engine. Some may regret the passing of a calm and peaceful way of life and the carving up of our beautiful countryside to allow access to this ubiquitous monster. But there are other drawbacks to this mode of transport, concerning health. It is now a major, if not *the* major, source of environmental chemical pollution. Some countries have vigorous laws to control emissions, but in the UK to date we have none.

In the meantime, chemically sensitive patients are left with a considerable problem.

If you must own and use a car, there are certain things you need to know. Firstly, the inside of the car itself is a source of many chemicals. Most of the fittings are plastic and give off fumes. The same is true of the upholstery. This is quite apart from any seepage of petrol odour into the cabin space. New cars are the worst and I have on a number of occasions had a patient swap their lovely gleaming new model with a friend who drives an older car (to the delight of the friend, of course). It takes several years for these odours to die away to a 'safe' level (for some patients, of course, there is no safe level), but in practical terms a new car becomes useable by all but the most sensitive patient after about six months.

Hot weather causes a great increase in the fumes from the vehicle interior as the fittings heat up. Thus a car could become worse as it gets older if this coincides with a period of higher ambient temperatures. If you notice you are worse after car journeys, especially on a hot day in a new car, this may be your problem.

Unfortunately, buying old cars also has its difficulties. Deterioration in the general condition of the vehicle may give rise to serious leaks of exhaust fumes which will themselves adversely affect the chemically sensitive occupant. Thus the only safe course is to purchase cars two to three years old and dispose of them by the time they are five or more years old. In any case, take a long drive in any car before you consider buying it and make sure that you can detect no significant odour.

Always keep the boot closed and do not travel with the hatchback open (as for carrying large items); this sucks in exhaust fumes to a serious level, enough to cause carbon monoxide poisoning.

Sublingual neutralising drops for hydrocarbon sensitivity may help, where you can obtain these from a practising clinical ecologist. If not, your best chance is to take large doses of vitamin C (four to twenty grammes depending on your tolerance) before and during your journey. Even this is useless if you are allergic to ascorbic acid (often manufactured from corn).

MOULDS

One of the most underdiagnosed group of allergens are the moulds. Yet these can account for an extraordinary diversity of symptoms, from indigestion to frank psychosis, as well as the obvious and well-known effects on the respiratory system. Dr Marshal Mandell of Norwalk, Connecticut has some startling videos of patients with bizarre symptoms under the influence of everyday moulds. Dr David Morris of Lacrosse, Wisconsin reported to fellow clinical ecologists recently (1984) that of 1,000 patients tested and treated for mould sensitivity (using the provocation-neutralisation method), almost all showed significant reaction to moulds and over ninety per cent were helped by this approach.

Moulds, by virtue of sporing, are in effect like all-year round pollen. Only in cold dry weather, such as on snowy or frosty days is the air really free of them. In older houses they abound and grow freely in the damp of wallpapers, carpets and fabrics, where liquids may have been spilled. Dry rot is simply another mould.

They are found too on our foods. Stored grains are especially susceptible but also other crops such as peanuts. Aflatoxin, a highly carcinogenic mould-produced poison which we may eat inadvertently when it is present in our food, is currently attracting much interest and there is great debate as to how we can best protect ourselves from this sort of ecological danger. It is estimated that, currently, twenty-five per cent of the world's food supply is being lost because of moulds (necessitating crop destruction).

On a historical note, contamination of rye by the mould ergot has been in the past responsible for frightening afflictions. It produces many highly poisonous substances (including LSD!) which typically cause madness and severe skin irritation. In mediaeval times, when rye was consumed as a bread staple, outbreaks of ergot poisoning were common and because they could not explain it people took it as a sign of God's wrath and called the attacks 'Holy Fire', (or St Anthony's fire).

It would be prudent to do as much as possible to avoid contact with moulds. If you live in an older house, it might be time for a move to a newer property. If you can't leave, check for and eradicate damp wherever possible (faulty guttering, leaking

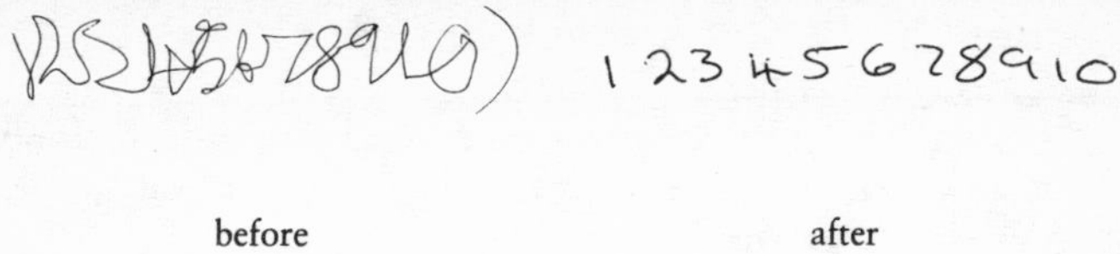

Fig. 8 *Example of handwriting deterioration while testing mould*

flashes etc). It can be expensive but in any case money spent in this way will usually enhance the value of your property. Check under carpets, under sinks (a favourite spot), along blinds, old fabrics etc. for signs of mould. Clear up what you find but put right the reason it was growing there in the first place.

A more drastic attack on the problem using formaldehyde as a fungicide is as follows:

Seal up all doors and windows so there are no draughts, place a small dish with about three ounces of formaldehyde (about fifty per cent strength) in each room, including the hallways and cellars and then leave the house for several days. If you are sensitive to formaldehyde, get someone else to do this for you. On return, they should also enter the building first, flush away all the formaldehyde and let fresh air circulate, possibly for several hours, before you allow yourself to go inside. Remember this is a hazardous procedure and take all due precautions.

PAINTS

Gloss paint is a powerful agent, causing unpleasant symptoms for many. If this applies to you, suspect chemical allergies in general. Avoid it if you can and do remember it gives off fumes for weeks afterwards.

Latex paint is said to be best. Stir in sodium bicarbonate until the paint stops bubbling (Markarness suggests about 500 grammes to five litres of paint).

SALT (sodium chloride)

I am often asked about allergy to salt. Even allowing for the liberal definition of allergy given on page 28 it is hard to reckon with an allergy to salt as such. However salt is a potentially harmful commodity and there is abundant evidence that it is connected with heart disease and hypertension, reason enough one would say to avoid it.

It is sometimes said that there is ample salt in food. I doubt this is true – even animals have salt licks – and modest supplementation is permissible.

But the way I see it you should not add salt during the cooking process *and* at the table. Do one or the other only. If you have a taste for salty food, this can be almost as harmful as a sweet tooth and you should work at getting rid of it.

TOOTHPASTE

Toothpaste is an allergist's nightmare. It often gets forgotten in exclusions and can lead to difficulties.

The trouble is it usually contains corn, sugar, colourings and potent allergens such as hexachlorophene and formaldehyde.

WELEDA (Ilkeston, Derbyshire) do a simple salt gel paste, which is safer than any other. For the exquisitely sensitive, try oil of cloves.

Epilogue

Last but not least ...
Perhaps some of it is in the mind!

In many ways, although short, this is one of the most important chapters in the book. Perhaps it would have been better to put it first but, as you will see, that isn't entirely logical either. The advice it contains should be taken seriously and is as important to you as all the technical and scientific information you have absorbed through these pages.

It is natural, when you are ill, to have your attention focused heavily on your body problem. It could hardly be otherwise. But it is vital that you consciously try to combat this tendency and don't allow yourself to become too introverted. As you have been reading, many allergy symptoms are vague and difficult to pin down. In fact it is possible to imagine any number of symptoms by thinking hard about different parts of your body. Yes I did say imagine. If you don't believe me, get a friend to concentrate hard on one part of their body. Ask them to report any feeling or sensation they may notice; nine times out of ten a symptom, however mild, will eventually appear. These would of course have no real validity in disease and I'm sure it's not being unkindly or hard-hearted to say such symptoms are not really unpleasant in the same way that true medical symptoms are.

This does not mean that I am coming round in a circle to the old 'all in the mind' theory, though in a way I am. A person's attitude to their illness is all important in the ability to conquer it. If you have an allergy and tackle it, with help, along the lines described in this book, staying optimistic and being willing to go through the vicissitudes of seeking and undergoing a cure, you should do well. Such an individual makes light of suffering and usually experiences a great deal of relief from simple remedies and minimum data. On the other hand, if you become fixated with your problems and always have something to complain about, forgetting the progress you have made and dwelling only on the negative aspects of your condition, the chances are your recovery will be limited.

I have seen many patients over the years and have been struck by the consistency of the above observation. Sometimes two people with seemingly identical diseases and similar allergies emerge from their treatments with completely different results. True enough, you may argue that each person is innately constitutionally unique and that explains the variation. But what I am reporting to you, without being able to give any statistics, for emotion is such an undefinable quantity, is my conviction that the cheerless and complaining souls are generally the ones that do badly and the happy and determined ones do better. In other words, it's a significant correlation that must mean something but which none of us so far can put into words (or useful methodology). What I'm saying is *think about something else*!

Take up a hobby, anything sensible; just get your mind off your illness. Going for long walks in the country (if you are able) may not be an allergy cure, but it is a *remedy* of sorts. Exercise, good company and social pleasures have their own rewards and do bring about a positive attitude towards life, health and human experience.

DON'T BECOME A HERMIT!

Because, by the nature of the illness, allergics have to avoid certain substances which are common in our environment, there is a constant pressure to shun human company and remain separated from others. Far too often patients find perfumes, cigarette smoke etc. have such dire consequences that they prefer to stay at home. This is wrong, no matter how tempting. The individual experiencing this plight often becomes highly introverted and so plunged even more deeply into an obsession with their condition, which is directly opposed to the advice given above and makes the problem, if such a thing is imaginable, far worse.

The loneliness and sense of frustrated isolation these patients experience is made more profound by the fact that few people at the time of writing really understand the nature of the problem and sympathy is lacking where it would be most appropriate. There is a tendency to look askance at allergics and treat them as freaks, an unfortunate state of affairs made worse by ignorance and misinformation within the medical profession. Let's face it, most people don't even believe in allergies, except the obvious ones like dust and strawberries, and this fuels the suspicion that allergic individuals are somehow not normal and therefore not nice. I'm pleased to say that the climate has changed recently, thanks to increasing media coverage, though even that, by its foolish and ephemeral nature, tends to dwell on the startling and unusual cases without seeking an understanding, which again reinforces prejudice against something seen as freaky.

You must make a positive effort (and it may be an effort) to contact others and share in a normal life-style. This is especially true for children, who certainly do not want to grow up feeling peculiar or 'different'. Be willing to take a few rebuffs; you will surely get some. But without being over optimistic, I think it is possible to state that most people have now heard of someone or other who is allergic and has to follow unusual restrictions on their lifestyle. Thus the strangeness of this 'strange disease' is growing less all the time, and this trend will continue due to increasing familiarity. See yourself, if you wish, as a pioneer, from whom others can learn, rather than as a curiosity. It all comes under thinking positively!

GET INVOLVED IN YOUR TREATMENT

It is almost contradictory to what I have just been saying to suggest that you take an active part in your treatment. Actually it isn't; this is all part of saying your attitude in tackling it will affect your ability to conquer your illness.

It isn't good enough to leave everything to the doctor. Even though clinical ecologists spend many hours with each patient, spread over many weeks, it is simply not possible to learn all there is to know about an individual. You, on the other hand, know more than anyone. You are present all the time, whatever your state of health and whenever you react to something. Thus you are the best possible observer of your own condition.

Clinical ecologists know this and are always willing to listen to what *you* have to say about your condition. A sad contrast, I'm afraid, with the normal approach of the medical profession.

It is vital that you learn as much as possible about allergies and their manifestations, in order that you can sensibly interpret what is happening to you. Again, clinical ecologists encourage this interest. We *like* our patients to know and understand their condition and abhor the all-too-common attitude of 'you're too dumb to understand'.

But you must balance this acquisition of knowledge against the problem of letting yourself become totally ruled by what you have learned. Even if you suffer with severe and widespread intolerances; everything that is happening to you is not explicable in terms of allergies!

STRESS

It would not be possible to touch on the subject of attitude of mind in illness without talking about stress. Remember, when I say this, that not all stress is mental. Any chronic illness, such as infections and malnutrition, is stressful; exhaustion and excessive physical exertion are similarly so. These factors can all make allergies worse by lowering the body's resistance. Allergies themselves are stressful, which is rather a vicious circle in some cases and explains why sometimes a patient gets ill due, say, to a virus condition and then never really gets over it (see post-viral fatigue syndrome, page 23). The allergies *themselves* maintain the stress and recovery is not possible until the allergies are detected and defused.

But mental stress is a reality. In our day and age it is one of the prime factors we have to contend with on health and disease. Yet, ironically, we know so little about it. It is even hard to define stress at times: what is stimulating and challenging on one occasion may some other time catch us in serious trouble and prove to be taxing and exhausting to the point of infirmity.

Hans Selye's theory about stress (Chapter 2) is a good one, in that it explains the observed facts and enables us to make certain predictions. For example, if stress goes on too long there will come a time when no adverse effects can be observed (stage 2) yet this will inevitably lead to a serious deterioration, unless the stress is removed (stage 3), the actual time interval varying according to the individual and the type of stress.

The bottom line of this is that allergics must avoid stress. If that sounds too perfect then let us say unnecessary stress or perhaps, even more exactly, that allergics should learn to contend with stress. It may not be possible to avoid a stressful experience (unless one wants to adopt the 'hermit' attitude referred to above) but if the patient can make an allowance for it, *by reducing stress in some other area*, the effects may not be so disastrous. Thus I often find myself, faced with a patient whose illness has returned during times of crisis, suggesting they revert to a much simpler and safer diet for a period. The rationale is that foods themselves may be stressful and those which are tolerated barely under optimum conditions are best avoided until the danger has passed. Going to bed to rest more may have the same effect (not to be encouraged too often). Other ways of reducing stress in a compensatory way may suggest themselves in individual cases. This is what I mean by learning to contend with stress, as opposed to merely avoiding it.

GET OUT OF THE FAST LANE

A lot of people ask for trouble by pushing themselves too far. It's a hectic society we live in today and often relentless pressure assails the individual who wants to do a little more than just get by. Success comes at a price and often the price is too high. It isn't really worth striving for material goals if by the time you achieve what you want bad health prevents you from enjoying your triumph. The neurotic rich are a study in hang-ups and pathology. It is worthwhile stopping to consider whether you really want to join them!

Remember, the body begins to recover as soon as you remove stress. It may take a long time but as soon as you control the adverse factors, things will begin to look up. The fact is it's never too late to change. There are many worthwhile goals in life, apart from a bigger mortgage or a prestigious car. It may be time to set yourself some spiritual goals; perhaps more time with the kids, that special holiday you've always promised yourself. Remember, the harder it is for you to contemplate this sort of thing, the more in the grip of the race you are. People who can take time off at the drop of a hat and go for a few days walking tour in Scotland are not really under much pressure. It is people who can't get away who are the ones who *must* do so, for their own good!

Perhaps you are not doing what you most want to do in life. This can build up into an unbearable stress and is a cause of a great deal of bitterness and frustration. A reappraisal of your career may be in order. The truth is many people have switched tracks successfully later in life and been glad they did. Neither is being sacked the end of the world, if the struggle to hold down a job is an unequal one. For some, any change would be an improvement and lead to a more worthwhile and contented way of life.

PSYCHOTHERAPY

Meditation, hypnotism and other forms of psychotherapy could be viewed as possible allergy treatments but in fact I have expressly excluded them in this overview. However they are certainly relevant to the subject of stress and I would simply say try them if you feel inclined.

There is no doubt that stressful events *from the past* can cause or prolong a current illness. We use a rather special form of stress release in my clinic and on many, many occasions taking the sting out of an unpleasant period in the patient's history has led to a remarkable recovery of the ability to tolerate foods and chemicals. Often such periods of stress immediately preceded the onset of the illness, or perhaps it was decades before and the bad feelings stay locked up in the mind, with dire consequences for the victim, until someone mercifully lets it out.

We have a lot to learn about the mind. Psychiatry has spent decades obscuring the real facts with erudite-sounding terminology and obfuscating ideas which have led to no useful advance in treatments and, in many cases, quite the reverse. I'm sure that the ultimate answers to disease lie even beyond 'the mind' in realms which might be called the spirit or life force.

THE ENERGY OF LIFE

Researchers from the UK and Russia have discovered that the body is surrounded by an electro-magnetic force field, which can actually be 'sensed' by some people and manipulated by sensitive healers.

It seems that life energy, that subtle and mysterious force which separates us from dead meat and inanimate forms, does indeed have physical properties. It seems rather to resemble a 'ghost' shell enveloping the body, possibly several layers thick. Disturbances in the equilibrium of these energy levels are apparently capable of causing illness and may be at the root of allergic disorders (recall that the auriculo-cardiac reflex method of testing for allergies (Chapter 6) operates by merely bringing the food or other test substances into the body's force field, without actually touching the skin).

Russian biophysicists report that a single human cell emits radio waves, hydrodynamic plasma waves, invisible waves close to the frequency of light and infrasonic acoustic waves. Obviously oriental mystics, sufis and the like were onto something centuries ago that modern science is only just beginning to catch up with. Remember we are composed of over 50 billion such cells: quite an orchestra!

The sun is by far the greatest source of electromagnetic radiation to which we are exposed. But it is estimated that we are now assaulted by some 200 million times the radiation levels our animal forebears had to endure, from radio and TV transmissions, telephones, microwaves, X-rays, computers. . . .

It would be surprising if this too was not having its adverse influence, in the same way that chemical deterioration in our environment is. (See also Chapter 10, p. 174 Electro-magnetic Fields.)

LAST WORD

There is much more to be learned. In some ways our present age resembles the last century or the Renaissance, such a great surge of human knowledge and endeavour is taking place. It is all rather exciting and it is a great thrill to be part of these advances.

So finally, I close by saying it really is *not* all in the mind. It is simply that thought and physics are finally meeting. Not before time, some might say!

Good luck.

Appendix 1

Total daily intake of a balanced nutritional programme

The following table contains recommendations for a balanced nutritional supplement from the book *Trace Elements, Hair Analysis and Nutrition* by Passwater and Cranton. Ideally these should be taken early in the morning before breakfast, or at night, so that excess quantities of a single element do not interfere with the absorption of other essential nutrients contained in meals.

Vitamin A (fish liver oil)	25,000 IU
Vitamin D (fish liver oil)	100 IU
Vitamin C (ascorbic acid)	1200 mgm
Vitamin B1 (thiamine HCl)	100 mgm
Vitamin B2 (riboflavine)	50 mgm
Vitamin B6 (pyridoxin HCl)	100 mgm
Vitamin B12	100 mcg
Niacin (nicotinic acid, B3)	50 mgm
Niacinamide (B3)	150 mgm
Pantothenic acid	500 mgm
Folic acid	800 mcg
Biotin	100 mcg
Choline	50 mgm
Inositol	100 mgm
PABA	50 mgm
Vitamin E (d-alpha-tocopheryl acetate)	400 IU
Calcium	500 mgm
Magnesium	500 mgm
Potassium	99 mgm

Iron	20 mgm
Iodine	250 mcg
Copper	2 mgm
Manganese	20 mgm
Zinc	20 mgm
Molybdenum	100 mcg
Chromium	200 mcg
Selenium	200 mcg
Bioflavinoids (rutin, hesperidine)	100 mgm
Trace minerals (ocean grown sources)	100 mgm

At present no single formula exists exactly duplicating the above quantities. However a number are available which are similar and by combinations of such it is possible to take the above quantities without needing dozens of tablets per day, which for allergics carries the additional risk of reacting to the bases in which the tablets are formulated.

Try to get those without sugar, starch, cereals or colouring additives. These are available. It may simply be a question of shopping around.

Appendix 2

*Chemical contamination**

THINGS CAUSING INDOOR CHEMICAL AIR CONTAMINATIONS

Eliminate as many as possible to reduce and eliminate your chemical sensitivity problems.

I. Fuels: Use electric heat and cooking. Avoid hydrocarbons, i.e. kerosene, coal, oil, gas, wood.
   1. These should not be in your garage if attached.
   2. Gas appliances must be removed. Won't help if only disconnected.
   3. If heating is electric, remove motor driven fans. These utilise oil. Use cool electric heat in form of radiator or heat pump installation – two stage controls of baseboard.
   4. Be sure there are no plastics in the heating ducts.
   5. Be sure filters are not oiled.
   6. Electronic filters dry dust and can give out dangerous gases.
   7 Use activated carbon filters.
   8. Be sure refrigerator has no leaks.

II. Avoid fresh paint and varnish and wood stain. Paint must be non-odorous. Casein paint is best. Use no rubber base paint.

* This appendix is taken from work published by Dr William Rea, of Dallas, Texas and reproduced here by kind permission of the author.

III. Avoid cements and other adhesives such as the following:
1. Finger nail polish and polish remover.
2. Shoe polish.
3. Paint remover.
4. Hinge looseners.
5. Adhesives used in model airplanes and other toys.
6. Adhesives containing tars for floors are very troublesome.

IV. Avoid cleaner and lighter fluids:
1. Be absent for several days if rags are cleaned.
2. Clothes should be aerated in the sun after being sent to dry cleaners.
3. No lighter fluids in the house

V. Newsprint: Newspapers and magazines should be opened and read by someone else first.

VI. Alcohol:
1. No rubbing alcohol.
2. No shellac, brush cleaning preparations.
3. Flavoring extracts have alcohol in them.

VII. Refrigerants and spray containers:
1. Slow escape of gas from refrigerators or air conditioners can cause trouble.
2. Same type gas is commonly used propellant in spray containers of insecticides, perfumes, hair sprays, and other cosmetics.

VIII. Insecticides:
1. DDT and related compounds are usually dispensed in kerosene and other solvents.
2. Avoid lindane, methoxychlor, DDT, chlordane, malathion, or thiocyanates.
3. Rugs are often moth proofed with fluids containing DDT while in storage. Rug shampoo can contain DDT.
4. Exterminators use dieldrin, chlordane, pentachloraphenol.
5. Blankets are often moth proofed similarly.
6. Moth balls, cakes, crystals containing naphthalene para-dichlorabenzene can cause symptoms.

IX. Sponge rubber:

1. Odours can come from sponge rubber pillows, mattresses, upholstery, rug pads, seat cushions, typewriter pads, rubber backing of rugs and various noise reducing installations.
2. Look out if one has restlessness, insomnia, night sweats, etc.

X. Plastics: The more flexible and odorous a plastic the more frequently it contributes to indoor chemical air pollution. Hard plastics like vinyl, Formica, bakelite, cellulose acetate . . . are rarely incriminated.

1. Vinyl and radiant floor heating fumes should be avoided.
2. Plastic pillows, combs, powder cases, shoes can give symptoms.
3. Avoid plastic air conditioning ducts.

XI. Mechanical devices:

1. Evaporating oil from any motor.
2. Air filters of glass wool or fibreglass usually have oiled filters, but one can get them without.
3. Fans and motors in hot water units.
4. Small kitchens may have too many motors.
5. Cars in garages or near elevator shafts can volatize gases.

XII. Miscellaneous:

1. Toxic fumes and odours can come from detergents, naptha-containing soaps, ammonia, chlorox, cleansing powders containing bleaches, some silver and brass polishing materials.
2. Storage of bleach containing cleansers.
3. Highly scented soaps, toilet deodorants, disinfectants – especially pine scented, air improvers.
4. Phenol and other chemicals are sometimes placed in wallpaper paste.
5. Pine Christmas trees, pine in wood burning fireplaces, creosote odours.
6. Odours from prolonged use of TV sets.

CHEMICAL CONTAMINATION OF INGESTANTS

A. A food additive is any chemical substance that makes its way into foods.

B. Susceptibility to chemical additives and contaminants of the diet has long been confused with specific susceptibility of [to] foods.

C. One may be sensitive to the food or the additive or both.

D. If one eats a food at one time and has no reaction, and then eats it another time and has a reaction, he probably is sensitive to the chemical and not the food.

E. Foods commonly contaminated by chemicals:

I. Foods often containing spray residues:

a. Apple, cherry, peach, apricot, nectarine, pear, plum, olive, currant, persimmon, strawberry, cranberry, raspberry, blueberry, boysenberry, pineapple, rhubarb, grape, orange, grapefruit, lemon.

b. Brussels sprouts, broccoli, cauliflower, cabbage, head lettuce, tomato, celery, asparagus, spinach, beet greens, chard, mustard greens, endive, escarole, leaf lettuce, romaine lettuce, chinese cabbage, artichoke.

1. Most commonly used sprays permeate the food to which they are applied.
2. They are not removed by washing, peeling, soaking in water or vinegar, or by cooking.
3. Root vegetables are apt to be free of spray residues unless contaminated in transit or in the market.

c. Lamb, beef, pork, fowl may be contaminated by the animals having eaten sprayed forage and concentrating such oil soluble insecticides, herbicides, or their vehicles in their fats. Chicken and turkey often contain residues of stilbesterol, a synthetic hormone.

II. Foods often containing fumigant residues: dates, figs, shelled nuts, raisins, prunes and other dried fruits, wheat, corn, barley, rice, dried peas, lentils.

III. Foods often containing bleaches: white flour (unbleached flour is usually available). Freshly stone-ground whole wheat flour is much safer.

IV. Foods often treated with sulphur:

a. Peaches, apricots, nectarines – often dusted with sulphur.

b. Commercially prepared fresh apples, peaches, apricots, and french fried potatoes may be treated with sulphur dioxide as an anti-browning agent.
c. Molasses, dried fruit, melon, citrus candied peel, and fruit marmalade may be bleached with sulphur dioxide.
d. Dried apple, dried pear, dried peach, dried apricot, raisin, prune, corn syrup (glucose), corn sugar (dextrose), cornstarch, corn oil usually are treated with sulphur dioxide in the process of manufacture.

V. Foods artificially coloured.
a. Crême de menthe, maraschino cherries and other coloured fruit, jello and other coloured gelatin desserts, mint sauce, coloured ice cream, coloured sherbert, coloured candy, coloured cake, cookie and pie frostings and fillings.
b. Weiners, bologna, cheese, butter, oleomargarine.
c. Orange, sweet potato, Irish potato.
d. Root beer, pop, cola drinks, and certain other soft and imitation drinks usually contain coal-tar dyes.

VI. Foods artificially sweetened: any containing saccharine or Sucaryl (sodium cyclamate).

VII. Foods exposed to gas:
a. Bananas are artificially ripened by exposure to ethylene gas.
b. Apple and pear are often stored in ethylene gas.
c. Coffee is often roasted over an open gas flame and may absorb some of the combustion products of such a flame.
d. Cane and beet sugars usually are clarified by being filtered through bone char. These filters are usually reactivated periodically in gas-fired kilns. Absorbed combustion products apparently are imparted to the next batch of syrup which is filtered through them.

VIII. Foods contaminated by containers:
a. Carrot, parsnip, turnip, tomato and mixed shredded greens dispensed in odorous plastic bags.
b. Certain other foods may also be contaminated by having been transported, stored, or frozen in plastic containers.

c. Cellophane wrapped foodstuffs are usually tolerated by chemically susceptible patients.
d. In general, plastic wrappings tend to contaminate their food contents in direct proportion to the odour emitted by the wrapping material.
e. The longer a food remains in an odorous plastic wrapping, the more it may be contaminated.
f. Plastic refrigerator dishes for storage of foods are commonly incriminated.
g. Citrus fruits may be contaminated by fungicide treated containers.
h. Foods are frequently contaminated by the golden brown lining of metal cans. This is a phenolic resin which prevents the metal from bleaching the contents of the can, but also contaminates them chemically. Only such foods as the manufacturer desires to bleach, such as asparagus, grapefruit, pineapple, artichoke, and some citrus juices, are apt to be packed in unlined cans.

IX. Foods often waxed with paraffin:
a. Rutabaga, parsnip, turnip, peppers, cucumber, eggplant, green pepper – waxed and lightly polished.
b. Apple, orange, grapefruit, tangerine, lemon – waxed and/or polished.

X. Foods often containing desiccating agents: prepared coconut – often contain added glycols.

XI. *Foods that are less chemically contaminated*:
a. *Fish and Meat* – fresh or frozen seafood (lobster, crayfish, shrimp, crab, etc.). Fresh fish or fish which has been frozen in large pieces (in contrast to pound packages) are not usually contaminated. Lean meat from which the fat has been stripped prior to cooking is preferable to cooking meat with its adherent fat.
b. *Vegetables* – fresh potato if undyed and home peeled, turnip, rutabaga, eggplant, parsnip (if not waxed), squash, pumpkin, beet (tops are usually sprayed), salsify, celery root, parsley root, okra, green peas, green beans (if fresh or canned in glass).
c. *Nuts* – nuts in shell only (Brazil nut, coconut, walnut, hickory nut, pecan, filbert, hazelnut).

d. *Sweetening agents* – honey, sorghum, *pure* maple sugar or syrup.

e. *Fats and Oils* – olive, cottonseed, peanut, soy, coconut, sunflower, sesame, safflower – preferably cold-pressed rather than extracted by the usual solvent process, buckwheat.

Importations such as chocolate, arrowroot, tapioca, carob and sassafras tea usually have been fumigated in shiphold.

Any food may have been contaminated in transit or in markets by sprayed surroundings in contaminated bulk cartons, plastic bags, or DDT treated burlap bags.

d. *Uncontaminated Food Sources* – Foods from approved local sources should be secured for canning in glass or freezing in glass or aluminium foil during the season of availability.

Membership in state or local Natural Food Associate groups or Organic Gardening Clubs is helpful in finding sources of supply.

This appendix is taken from work published by Dr William Rea of Dallas, Texas and reproduced here by kind permission of the author.

Appendix 3

List of useful names and addresses

Several groups and organisations are mentioned in the text. Contact addresses are given below. Others are included as groups of environmental interest.
Note: I do not endorse the activities of any of these groups, except ACTION AGAINST ALLERGY. They are merely included as worthy of note. You must satisfy yourself of their usefulness and sincerity.

Action Against Allergy (AAA)
43 The Downs,
London SW20 8HG
(01) 947 5082

Aims: To make the problems of allergy sufferers known and to disseminate information and technical data regarding allergies to the public and medical profession alike.

Activities: Lectures, broadcasts and film shows. Runs a comprehensive information service and library for use by doctors. Supports research. Sells books.

National Society for Research into Allergy
P.O.Box 45
Hinckley
Leicestershire

Supports investigation into allergic phenomena and cures. A bit stuffy and very 'establishment'. One of their senior officials is quoted as saying she 'didn't believe in clinical ecology' and one of their research doctors said in my presence he was basically trying to prove that treatments are ineffective though how much tongue-in-cheek it is hard to say. In the context of this book you may find these remarks off-putting. Make up your own mind based on what you find.

British Medical Acupuncture Society (BMAS)
67–69 Chancery Lane,
London WC2 1AF

Aims To promote the use and scientific understanding of Acupuncture as part of the practice of medicine.

Activities: A society for medical practitioners only. Regular scientific meetings and teaching courses are held for doctors. Members are available to lecture to non-medical societies and the secretary will answer written enquiries from the public.

Publications: Acupuncture in Medicine (BMAS journal).

British Chiropractors' Association (BCA)
5 First Avenue,
Chelmsford
Essex CM1 1RX
024 58487/0423 870945

Aims: To regulate the activities of members. To promote the practice of chiropractice by qualified practitioners and to seek formal recognition of the profession.

Activities: Maintains a register of chiropractors who have graduated from recognised colleges and who subscribe to the Association's code of ethics, designed to protect the public interest. The Bye-Laws and Code of Ethics regulate relationships between chiropractors, patients and other members and practitioners.

Publications: Contact

British Ecological Society (BES)
Burlington House,
Piccadilly, London W1V OLQ
(01) 434 2641

Aims: To advance the education of the public and to advance and support research in the subject of ecology as a branch of natural science and to disseminate the results of such research.

Activities: Publishing; organising scientific meetings and symposia; supporting research and training.

Publications: Journal of Ecology; Journal of Animal Ecology; Journal of Applied Ecology.

British Holistic Medical Association
23 Harley House,
Marylebone Road,
London NW1 5HE
(01) 487 4227

Aims: The education of doctors, medical students and allied professions to the principles and practice of holistic medicine. To inform the general public; to act as a resource for like-minded bodies; to encourage research studies and publish relevant material; to provide liaison between fellow practitioners for mutual support and personal and professional development.

Activities: Regular conferences, workshops and lectures; production of journal and news bulletins; will be setting up local branches.

Publications: Journal of the BHMA

British Nutrition Foundation (BNF)
15 Belgrave Square,
London SW1X 8PS
(01) 235 4904/9

Aims: To advance knowledge in nutrition and the education of the public in nutrition through research and the dissemination of information.

Activities: Publication of the bulletin, monographs and briefing papers; organisation of conferences and specialist meetings; promotion of research.

Status: Registered limited company recognised by the Charities Act.

Publications: BNF Nutrition Bulletin.

British Organic Farmers (BOF)
Leggatts Park,
Potters Bar,
Herts EN6 1NZ
0707 58561

Aims: A self help farmers group to promote contact between and disseminate information to farmers and others interested in organic food production, with a view to assisting them in improving production.

Activities: Farm walks; publication of journal; conferences; statistical information; forthcoming soil analysis service.

Publication: The New Farmer and Grower.

British Touch for Health Association (BTFHA)
29 Bushey Close,
High Wycombe,
Bucks
0494 37409

Activities: Courses in Touch for Health (based on Applied Kinesiology), a wonderful tool for all practitioners, to be used in conjunction with their own skills, for stress and anxiety states, dietary and allergy testing and structural balancing using simple muscle testing and touch correction.

Publication: Newsletter.

Conservation Trust
c/o George Palmer School,
Northumberland Avenue,
Reading, Berks.
RG2 OEN
0734 868442

Aims: To encourage greater environmental awareness amongst people of all ages.

Activities: Information service on environmental topics.

Resource bank of teaching materials, including books, slides, posters, etc., available on free loan to members. Publications, mainly relating to environmental education, include series of study notes, guides and packs (large s.a.e. with inquiries).

Publications: Newsletter; Guide to Resources in Environmental Education; Environmental Education Enquiries.

Department of the Environment (DoE)
2 Marsham Street,
London
SW1P 3EB
(01) 212 3434

Activities: The Secretary of State is responsible for strategic issues of expenditure and the financial, economic and environmental impact of policy. The Minister for Local Government and Environmental Services is responsible for local government, land use and development, minerals, countryside, inner areas, regional affairs, water and environmental protection. The Minister for Housing and Construction is responsible for housing construction, new towns, Property Services Agency, conservation, historic buildings and monuments and royal parks and palaces. Several parliamentary under-secretaries of state share responsibilities for assisting ministers and for other duties such as energy conservation or noise.

The department controls a number of Directorates and Units and has various research establishments, including the Transport and Road Research Laboratory, the Building Research Establishment and the Hydraulics Research Station. The Central Unit on Environmental Pollution has a general co-ordinating role, usually undertakes UK representation at international meetings and can direct inquiries to suitable specialists. The department shares some common services with the Department of Transport.

The library produces several regular publications and bibliographies.

Ecology Party (ECO)
36–38 Clapham Road,
London SW9 OJQ
(01) 735 2485

Aims: A democratic party whose policies are based on the principle that people must live in harmony with nature within the limitations of the Earth's finite supply of resources.

Activities: Fighting elections at local, national and European level. Campaigning on environmental, peace and economic issues. Raising public consciousness of 'green politics' and the need for a sustainable no-growth economy. Branches throughout the UK.

Publication: Econews

E.M.A.S. Advisory Service
1 Chepstow Place,
Westbourne Grove,
London W2 4TF
(01) 299 3456

Activities: Carries out research into problems in occupational medicine, including those resulting from air pollution, lead absorption, etc. Issues a series of Notes of Guidance on pollutants such as asbestos, cadmium, carbon dioxide, carbon mnonoxide, ionising radiations, lead, mercury, noise, selenium and vanadium.

Health & Safety Executive (HSE)
Regina House,
259 Old Marylebone Road,
London W1 5RR
(01) 723 1262

Activities: Comprises various Inspectorates, Branches, Divisions and Units responsible to the Health and Safety Commission. Reports on all areas of industrial health and safety, an example being the *Quarterly Statement on Nuclear Incidents*.

Henry Doubleday Research Association (HDRA)
20 Convent Lane,
Bocking,
Braintree,
Essex CM7 6RW
0376 24083

Aims: To improve and encourage agriculture and horticulture. To research and study improved methods of organic farming and gardening. To disseminate knowledge of the results of such research among farmers, gardeners and schools.

Activities: Maintaining a two-acre Trial Ground which is laid out to demonstrate organic gardening; conducting experiments; organic advice service (strictly members only); producing leaflets; supplying hard-to-buy materials; maintaining a specialist library.

Publications: Newsletter.

Institute for Complementary Medicine
21 Portland Place,
London W1N 3AF
(01) 636 9543

Aims: To promote natural therapeutics and methods of healing.

Medical Research Council
20 Park Crescent,
London W1N 4AL
(01) 636 5422

Environmental Hazards Unit: St Bartholomew's Hospital, Charterhouse Square, London EC1 6BQ (01) 235 1537

Environmental Radiation Unit: Department of Medical Physics, University of Leeds, W. Yorks 0532 31751

Toxicology Unit: Woodmansterne Road, Carshalton, Surrey SM5 4EF

Publications: Handbook

Organic Growers Association (OGA)
Aeron Park,
Llangeitho,
Tregaron,
Dyfed,
Wales
097423 272

Aims: To present the interests of organic fruit and vegetable growers; to provide a forum for discussion and mutual support; to educate the public about the benefits of organic agriculture.

Activities: Conferences; workshops; farm walks; special packaging for organic growers.

Publications: New Farmer and Grower

Soil Association
86–88 Colston Street
Bristol
BS1 5BB
0272-29066

Aims: To promote organic farming and discourage the indiscriminate use of persistent pesticides and artificial fertilisers.

Activities: Advising farmers who wish to know more about organic husbandry. Conducting courses in the principles and practice of organic husbandry. Demonstrating the advantages of organic methods through conferences, lectures and exhibitions. Sponsoring the marketing of organic produce. Promoting research and arranging field trials. Co-operating with other organisations in the ecological movement. Issuing a magazine and running a bookshop. Local groups.

Publications: Soil Association Journal

Touch for Health
1174 N. Lake Avenue
Pasadena
CA 91104
USA

Appendix 4

Auto-Immune Deficiency Syndrome (AIDS)

I have assigned these brief notes about AIDS to an appendix since I myself have not been personally involved with this disease. Nevertheless, it holds a great deal of interest for those who suffer with allergies. It seems fairly clear to me that there is a close resemblance between the presentation of AIDS and the symptoms so typical of allergy, as outlined earlier in the book. This similarity is so striking that many cases of AIDS will be missed, unless the physician is on the alert, as all doctors should be. It is equally probable that a number of allergy sufferers will be wrongly labelled as cases of AIDS, if their personal life happens to bring them under suspicion of contact.

In fact I'm prepared to stick my neck out and say that AIDS, a failure of the body's immunological defences, is on the increase for much the same reason that allergies are: we are poisoning ourselves and overloading this delicately balanced and sensitive immune mechanism within our bodies. This is not to say that AIDS isn't a viral disease and contagious but, as we saw in Chapter 1, even familiar viral infections such as influenza are able to damage the immunity system. But I believe it is important to consider if any environmental factors exist (such as pollution) to *predispose* this damage to take place. If I'm right and this does happen, this is a very important new view in the aetiology (origins and causes) of AIDS. It means we are in for a world-wide pandemic of AIDS.

DEFINITION

The definition used by the Communicable Disease Surveillance Centre at Colindale is the same as that in use at the Center for Disease Control in Atlanta, Georgia, USA:

1. A reliably diagnosed disease that is at least moderately indicative of an underlying cellular immune deficiency. For example, Kaposi's sarcoma in a patient aged less than 60 years, or opportunistic infection.
2. No known underlying cause of the cellular immune deficiency nor any other cause of reduced resistance reported to be associated with the disease.

Incidentally, this definition has been endorsed in many other countries and also by the WHO Collaborating Centre of AIDS.

TESTS

It is known that AIDS is transmitted by a virus (human T-lymphocytotropic virus – HTLV-III). At the time of writing, an antigen titre test is becoming available in the UK and doubtless, in due course, the definition above will be modified to include a raised titre as a part of the diagnostic criteria.

SYMPTOMS

Recognised symptoms make very interesting reading and some bear a striking resemblance to allergic disorders. It is possible, for example, to confuse AIDS with asthma, eczema and colitis, depending on what symptoms are in evidence. Intestinal thrush may be present (see page 25). But possibly the most important group of symptoms are the mental changes, which seem very like cerebral allergies. They may include lethargy, depression, confusion, fits, headaches, disorientation and loss of memory. Compare these with the table on page 8 and you will see why I am convinced there is a link between AIDS and maladaptation.

Glandular fever may be mimicked and this condition too is often easy to confuse with acute maladaptation episodes, except when laboratory tests come to the rescue

I have referred to AIDS, not to add to the scare-mongering, but because I think it can teach us something about allergic and environmental disease. Too little is known at present to be able to draw categorical conclusions, except that it is a sinister view of what is in store for us if indeed we are poisoning our defense mechanism. Whatever the social, infective and ecological factors that are relevant, the final pathway seems clear – impairment of our immunological systems bodies will have rapid and serious consequences for us all, AIDS or not.

If you have a chronic debilitating allergy-type illness, it would be wise to get your doctor to suggest a blood test for AIDS, which you are now entitled to do.

Appendix 5
Hyperventilation

The subject of hyperventilation is of considerable importance to many allergics. Yet I have had to consign it to an appendix; largely because very little useful scientific work has been published on this topic. To date it remains mainly a subject of discussion and exchange of views among interested doctors at seminars, dinners, conferences and such. But until more is learned, I do not see why the public should not be entitled to hear of it for themselves in the meantime.

Opinions seem to divide us into two distinct groups (a) those who believe that hyperventilation – and not allergies – is the real cause of the patient's symptoms and (b) those who think that allergies trigger hyperventilation, which then leads to symptoms, but that allergies come first.

I myself belong very firmly to the latter group and I think most allergists and clinical ecologists do likewise. In any case, nothing in this appendix is intended to suggest that allergies may not in fact exist and that it is all really a problem in breathing!

WHAT IS HYPERVENTILATION?

The word means over-breathing: that is, breathing in excess of physiological requirements.

In the normal course of events air is drawn into the lungs, oxygen is removed into the blood and, at the same time, carbon dioxide is given off as a waste product which appears in the exhaled breath. We call this process respiration or, more correctly *external respiration.* (Internal respiration is the combustion of foods with oxygen that takes place directly within the tissues under the regulating control of many enzymes.)

The uptake of oxygen need not concern us here. It is tightly bound to haemoglobin (the red blood pigment) and remains at a fairly constant level, provided the lungs are working normally.

Carbon dioxide, on the other hand, dissolves directly into the plasma. A simple chemical reaction takes place, which may be represented by the equation:

$$\underset{\text{carbon dioxide}}{CO_2} + \underset{\text{water}}{H_2O} = \underset{\text{carbonic acid}}{H_2CO_3}$$

Carbonic acid dissociates into $H+$ ions and HCO_3- (bicarbonate) ions and this affects the acidity of the blood (pH, for those with scientific knowledge).

Both the kidneys and the lungs control bicarbonate levels, the kidneys by selective extraction and the lungs by blowing off extra carbon dioxide. There are chemicals present in the blood called buffers which are able, to a certain extent, to mop up excess acidic and alkaline ions but there is a limit to how much compensation can take place this way, especially when something is wrong which is causing a chronic departure from the optimum acidity.

You will now readily see, I hope, that overbreathing will lower the carbon dioxide levels excessively, which will deplete blood bicarbonate and this in turn will upset the body's acid-base equilibrium enough to cause symptoms in susceptible patients.

Of course, we are talking about unconscious *involuntary* overbreathing now, not something indulged in temporarily in order to play the bagpipes or some similar act. It is a bad habit that has become elevated to the status of a disease process!

SYMPTOMS

The principal symptoms are due to effects on the brain, which is the organ most vulnerable to subtle biochemical changes of this sort. The two most typical symptoms are chronic fatigue and dizzyness. If the the dizzyness is pronounced and alarming, this can sometimes cause the patient to panic, which may make matters worse due to the panting respiration often associated with great apprehension or fear. A vicious circle is thus set up which may end up with the patient out cold in a dead faint, though fortunately it rarely becomes so extreme.

In my days as a medical student hyperventilation was thought to be nothing more than a problem of hysterical women and the cure was to get the patient to breathe in and out of a paper bag! Believe it or not, this is correct physiologically. R*e*-breathing the carbon dioxide just exhaled increases the blood levels and the situation corrects itself very rapidly. It is a very impressive demonstration for everyone – the onlookers, the patient and the wet-behind-the-ears medical student.

The only new discovery is really that this is a much wider problem than realised formerly and that it can cause many other deep-rooted problems, not just panic and trembling. Once again, it is worth emphasising that many of the symptoms listed in chapter 3 can be caused by hyperventilation, especially those attributable to the central nervous system.

TESTS

There are no tests to detect this problem, though serum potassium can be chronically low and is well worth checking.

The only real way to diagnose it for certain is for the patient deliberately to over-breathe by way of a test. This should be done with the individual lying down and preferably accompanied by someone who understands their condition. If the familiar group of symptoms appear, the diagnosis is obvious.

It is often a source of great satisfaction, and of course relief, to a distressed patient to find that the symptoms which have been troubling her so persistently and perhaps frighteningly are caused by nothing more than faulty breathing.

TREATMENT

Drug treatment is quite inappropriate though I see it as inevitable that some of my colleagues will want to tackle the problem this way.

The real answer lies in retraining the patient to breathe correctly. Help from an expert physiotherapist is invaluable in this but *beware*: most physiotherapists make the problem worse by teaching the patient how to breathe deeply and efficiently, which is fine for someone with asthma but the exact opposite of what is wanted here.

For some individuals, the only available help may be from yoga or a similar discipline, though again it must be stated that only teachers who know how to deal with hyperventilation should be consulted.

During severe panic attacks the old paper bag trick is as valid as ever. If the patient can be reasoned with get her (or him) to breathe out, count for six long seconds, then breathe in slowly, out again, hold for six more seconds, and so on. It should be possible to slow the respiration down to about ten per minute or less.

Glossary

Adenitis: inflammation of glands.

Adrenal glands (see endocrine glands): Situated above the kidney, these vital organs are responsible for secreting adrenalin in times of stress, also steroid hormones which help the body's immunity and defence mechanisms.

Aetiology: the factors contributing to the causation of an illness.

Agglutinate: to stick together, as in a test where this will only occur when certain antibodies are present.

Allergic extrinsic asthma: a kind of asthma classically associated with external stimuli such as dust and feathers.

Anaphylaxis: a sudden and violent allergy reaction in which there is circulatory collapse and which is often fatal.

Anorexia nervosa: a condition in which the patients' perception of their body image, in relation to food, is grossly distorted. They see themselves as fat whereas in fact they are thin, and try desperately to lose weight, even though they may be already dangerously underweight.

Aphasia: inability to speak.

Arteriosclerosis: hardening of the arteries.

arteritis: inflammation of arteries.

Arthralgia: pain in the joints from whatever cause (arthritis is the most common).

Aspergillosis: an infection with aspergillus, a pathogenic fungus which sometimes invades the lung and other tissues.

Asymptomatic: without symptoms.

Ataxia: inability to make correctly co-ordinated movements, or to walk evenly.

Atopic: Arthur Coca's original word for the person highly susceptible to classic allergic disorder, such as asthma, eczema, urticaria and rhinitis.

Atrophy: disintegration or wastage of tissue.

Autogenous: self-generating as from a cause within.

Basophils: white blood cells which stain with a basic dye.

Calcinosis: condition in which excess calcium is deposited in the tissues and where calcified patches can be seen on X-ray where they do not belong.

Candidiasis: an overgrowth of **candida albicans**, the organism causing thrush, which can become toxic due to causing bowel permeability.

Cardiovascular: having to do with the heart and blood vessel system.

Cerebral cortex: that part of the brain which contains the living nerve cells. It is grey in colour (grey matter). The cerebral hemispheres are where Man's higher thought functions are located.

Chelating agents: chemicals which bind with heavy metals in the blood. These are then passed out through the kidney, which is a way of removing unwanted poisonous metals such as lead and mercury.

Cocksackie: a kind of large virus.

Coeliac disease: condition in which the lining of the intestine is severely damaged by allergy to gluten, a protein found in certain cereals (wheat, rye, barley and oats). In its most extreme form the patient suffers malnutrition due to loss of vital foodstuffs which are unable to be absorbed.

Colitis: inflammation of the colon, characterised by recurring diarrhoea, blood and occasionally mucus.

Conjunctiva: membranous lining covering the eye which when kept moist protects it from damage and invasion by bacteria, dirt, etc.

Crohn's disease (regional ileitis): an inflammatory condition of the small bowel causing pain and diarrhoea which leads to damage and eventual death of bowel tissue.

Cutaneous: having to do with the skin.

Cystitis: inflammation of the bladder, mostly characterised by a frequent desire to pass urine and a scalding sensation in so doing.

Cytoplasm: principal ingredient inside a living cell (the other chief ingredient is the nucleus or nuclear protein).

Dander: dead skin scales (e.g. dandruff).

Dermatitis: any rash or irritation of the skin but most often reserved for conditions caused by external chemicals.

Dermographism: a condition associated with allergies in which slight pressure on the skin causes severe whealing. The name is derived from the fact that one can write one's name on the patient's back using light finger touch pressure; shortly afterwards the resultant wheals stand out clearly.

Dermatitis: any rash or irritation of the skin but most often reserved for conditions caused by external chemicals.

Endocrine glands: that group of glands, including the thyroid, sex glands and adrenals, which have their effect by secreting a chemical called a hormone directly into the bloodstream, which has its effect on a distant part of the body.

Enzymes: chemicals which facilitate chemical reactions which would otherwise not easily take place. Some are involved in digestion, e.g. lipase digests fat, but there are thousands of others present in cells and vital for their normal healthy functioning.

Exocrine glands: the opposite of endocrine glands. They secrete their liquids into a duct or tube which carries them to where they are required. e.g. the salivary gland is exocrine.

Fibroid (adjective): fibre-like tissue which changes into rough fibrous tissue instead of its normal functioning character.

Glomerular nephritis: an inflammatory process in the kidney. At least some cases have been identified as allergic in origin.

Glucuronidase: an enzyme which acts on glucuronic acid, an important constituent of chondroitin sulphate (found in cartilage) and hyaluronic acid (found in synovial fluid).

Haemolytic anaemia: those anaemias caused by damage, i.e. haemolysis of red blood cells.

Haemorrhagic necrosis: damage and destruction of tissue with bleeding present.

Histamine: one of a number of chemical substances released during a classical allergic reaction. It causes reddening and whealing of the skin and local irritations.

Holistic (occasionally spelt wholistic): regarding the body as a whole and entire organism not as individual parts.

Homeostasis: (see text) keeping everything stable physiologically (*homeo* = same).

Humoral: concerns the chemical relay of information as opposed to nervous tissue relay (see endocrine system).

Hyalase: an enzyme which dissolves hyalin, the transparent chemical which binds together cells and other tissues.

Hypertension: high blood pressure.

Hypoglycaemia: low blood sugar which can cause a diversity of symptoms, particularly including tiredness, irritability and urgent hunger. Often caused, ironically, by eating too many sweet foods.

Ige: immunoglobins, i.e. heavyweight proteins present in the blood and known to be associated with immunity are characterised by different numbers such as IgG and IgE.

Innervate: to supply with nerves.

Intradermal: within the skin, as opposed to hypodermic, under the skin.

Lupus-erythematosus: an auto-immune disease where antibodies attack a number of organs in the body and cause damage and serious illness.

Lymphocyte activity: lymphocytes are one type of white blood cells involved in the fight against infections and other disease processes. The helper and suppressor lymphocytes are present in any such activity and speed up or reduce the process to keep it in optimum balance. AIDS has its damaging effect apparently by causing excess of suppressors which lower immunity.

Lymphocyte response: in all inflammatory or infectious processes, white blood cells are mobilized to fight off the attack. Lymphocytes are one type of white cell. Monocytes, basophils, eosinophils are other types, which need not concern us here.

Manic: suffering from mania – extreme excitability, wild behaviour, often shouting and delirium; activity of an extreme degree (cf. hypomania which is a milder, less extreme, type of overstimulation).

Mast cells: are present in a wide variety of tissue, at times of allergic reaction or damage they break down and release histamine, which causes local swelling and inflammation.

Menière's disease: disease of inner ear which affects middle-aged people, particularly women, characterised by deafness and attacks of dizziness.

Minimata disease: mercury poisoning first observed in the bay of Minimata in Japan and caused by pollution affecting fish in the local bay. The two most striking features are muscular twitching and mental deterioration.

Monilia albicans: another name for *Candida albicans*, a yeast-like organism which causes thrush or candidiasis.

Morbidity: disease processes.

Multiple sclerosis (disseminated sclerosis): As yet this is a poorly understood condition, with widespread intermittent damage to nervous tissue, which can manifest itself in a number of ways, usually widespread and of no determinate pattern.

Myalgia: pain in the muscles.

Mycobacteria: a group of bacteria including the causative organisms for TB and leprosy.

Myositis: inflammation of the muscles.

Nephrotic syndrome: a condition which attacks the kidneys, characterised by copious volumes of urine containing excess protein.

Neuralgia: nerve pain.

Neurasthenia: a condition of extreme apathy and lethargy.

Neuromuscular transmission: the chemical process which transfers the electrical impulse passing down the nerve to the muscle and so causes the muscle to contract. Acetylchlorine is one of the chemicals involved in this process. It is interrupted by a number of chemicals including organo-phosphorus pesticides, which will thus cause paralysis.

Oedematous: puffiness due to fluid retention.

Oligo-antigenic: low in substances that are likely to cause allergies (an alternative is hypoallergenic as in hypoallergenic make-up).

Opportunistic infections: Those which would otherwise not take place were it not for the fact that the body's defences are undermined and weakened. Germs which normally occupy the throat causing little harm, for example, are able to invade the body causing severe inflammation and distress. *Candida albicans* can become an opportunistic infection if the individual is severely debilitated either by the frequent use of antibiotics, any chronic disease, contraceptive pill, or use of steroids. The crossover between allergic illness and AIDS in this respect is discussed in Appendix 4.

Paroxysmal tachycardia: a sudden attack of extremely fast heartbeat, upwards of 200 beats per minute. The individual experiences faintness and may pass out, since the heart at this rate cannot perform properly and the brain becomes starved of blood.

Pathogenesis: the causation of disease.

Peptic ulcer: any ulcer caused or influenced by the presence of stomach acid, chiefly of two types, gastric and duodenal ulcer. The allergic causation is often overlooked.

Pinna: the outer, visible part of the ear, the flap.

Polymyalgia rheumatica: a poorly understood condition, almost certainly of allergic nature in which there are widespread aches and pains attacking various parts of the body, usually muscles – hence polymyalgia.

Polymyositis: widespread inflammatory patches in the muscles which cause pain.

Pseudopodia: a Greek word meaning foot-like used to describe the protruberances made by microscopic cells when they are 'oozing' from one position to another.

Purpura: a condition which includes bruising and bleeding patches under the skin.

Rhinitis: inflammation of the nasal passages causing stuffiness and running nose, usually of an allergic nature.

Schizophrenia: this condition is extremely hard to define. Basically it is characterised by an extreme detachment from reality. A schizophrenic accepts distortions of reality that you and I would not – this may include hearing 'voices', or feeling 'rays' coming from a radio set, or delusions of being persecuted by other people (paranoia).

Sedimentation rate: the measure of how fast the red blood cells settle when the blood is left to stand. It is raised non-specifically in a number of conditions.

Septicaemia: a condition in which bacteria have invaded the blood and become widely disseminated. It is extremely serious and prior to antibiotics, almost invariably fatal.

Solar dermatitis: inflammation of the skin brought about by the sun's rays, hence 'allergic to the sun'. In reality the sun is merely a trigger and underlying allergies are usually the cause.

Spectroscopic analysis: obtained from an instrument used to split up light or other radiation into components of different wavelengths. The simplest spectroscope uses a prism, which splits white light into the rainbow colours of the visible spectrum.

Staphylococcus: a type of bacterium commonly found in the mouth or skin and often responsible for infections of cuts and wounds.

Sympathetic nervous system: part of the autonomic nervous system, the self-regulating part of the body's nervous tissues, responsible for such unconscious actions as bowel movement, glandular secretions, heart rate etc. It is divided into two parts, the sympathetic system which stimulates the body in a similar way to adrenalin, i.e. increased heart rate, perspiration, muscle tone and sphincter activity and the para sympathetic system, which has the opposite effect.

Syndrome: collection of symptoms forming an identifiable pattern. Colicky pains, peripheral nerve weakness and mental deterioration is a syndrome caused by lead poisoning.

Systemic lupus-erythematosis: an auto-immune disease where antibodies attack a number of organs in the body and cause widespread damage and serious illness.

Tinnitus: a ringing in the ears or any rasping irritating noise in the ears.

Titre: an amount of something measured by actual testing.

Urticaria: inflammatory rash caused by allergies, characterised by swelling and itching, not unlike the response to a stinging nettle (Latin *Urtica urens = nettle*).

Vacuolate: to turn into vacuoles, which are spaces. This occurs when a cell dies – hollow activities begin to appear in the cell.

Vasculitis: Inflammation of blood vessels.

Wilson's disease: inborn defect of copper metabolism in which there is a deficiency of caeruloplasmin (which normally forms a nontoxic complex with copper). The free copper may be deposited in the liver, causing jaundice and cirrhosis, or in the brain, causing mental retardation and symptoms resembling Parkinsonism.

References

Chapter 1

1. Coca, A. F., *Familial non-Reaginic Food Allergy* (Charles C. Thomas, Springfield, Illinois, 1953).
2. Mackarness, R., *Chemical Victims* (Pan Books, London, 1980).
3. Behan, P. O., Behan W. M. H. and Bell, E. J., 'The Postviral Fatigue Syndrome: An Analysis of the Findings in 50 Cases' (unpublished paper) reprints from P. O. Behan, Institute of Neurological Sciences, Southern General Hospital, 1345 Govan Road, Glasgow G5 4TF.
4. Businco, L., 'Chronic Influenza Disease: An Experimental Model of a New Pathology', in *Clinica Europa*, *Anno* XIX-*N5* (Rome, Sept.-Oct. 1980).
5. Crook, Dr W., *The Yeast Connection* (Professional Books, Jackson, Tennessee, 1983).
6. Ibid.

Chapter 2

1. Coombs, R. R. A. and Gell, P. G. H., *Clinical Aspects of Immunology* (Blackwell Scientific, Oxford, 1969) pp. 575–96.
2. Feingold, B. F., MD, *Introduction to Clinical Allergy* (Charles C. Thomas, Springfield, Illinois, 1973) p. 3.

3. Randolph, T. G., in *Clinical Ecology*, ed. Lawrence Dickey (Charles C. Thomas, Springfield, Illinois, 1976).
4. Ibid.
5. Finn, R. and Cohen, H. N., 'Food Allergy: Fact or Fiction?' in the *Lancet* (London, 25 Feb 1978).
6. Dickey, L., *Clinical Ecology* (Charles C. Thomas, Springfield, Illinois, 1976) p. 33.
7. Hamlyn, Dr E. C., Rutt House, Ivybridge, Devon (private monograph).
8 Soil Association, Walnut Tree Manor, Haughley, Stowmarket, Suffolk IP14 3RS, *Pall of Poison* (booklet) (1984).
9. Finn and Cohen, *op. cit.* pp. 426–8.
10. Jones, A. J. *et al.*, 'Food Intolerance: A Major Factor in the Pathogenesis of Irritable Bowel Syndrome', in the *Lancet* (London, Nov. 20 1982) pp. 1115–7.
11. Egger, J. *et al.*, 'Is Migraine Food Allergy?', in the *Lancet* (London, 15 Oct. 1983) pp. 865–8.
12. Ibid.

Chapter 3

1. Mandell, M., *Dr Mandell's 5-Day Allergy Relief System* (Growell, New York, 1979) pp. 84–8.
2. Randolph T. G. and Moss R. W., *Allergies: Your Hidden Enemy* (Thorsons, Wellingborough, 1981) p. 30.
3. Randolph, T. G., 'Stimulatory and Withdrawal Levels of Manifestations', in *Clinical Ecology* ed. Lawrence Dickey (Charles C. Thomas, Springfield, Illinois, 1978).

Chapter 4

1. Cornaro, L., *How to Live 100 Years* (Thorsons, Wellingborough, 1951).
2. Jones *et al.*, *op cit.* (see chap. 2, note 10).
3. Mackarness, R. 'Stone-Age Diet for Functional Disorders', in *Medical World*, 91 (London, 1959) pp. 14–19.
4. Rinkel, H. J., Randolph, T. G. and Zeller, M., *Food Allergy* (Charles C. Thomas, Springfield, Illinois, 1951).
5. Coca, A. F., *The Pulse Test* (ARC Books, New York, 1959).
6. Randolph, *op. cit.* (see chap. 3, note 2) p. 186.

Chapter 5

1. Blackley, C., *Experimental Researches in Catarrhus Aestivus* (Balliere, Tindal and Cox, London, 1873).
2. Schofield, A. T., 'A Case of Egg Poisoning', in the *Lancet*, 1 (London, 1908) p. 716.
3. Noon, L., 'Prophylactic Innoculation against Hay Fever', in the *Lancet*, 1 (London, 1911) p. 1572.
4. Rinkel *et al*, *op. cit* (see chap. 4, note 4) p. 170.
5. Feingold, *op. cit.* (see chap 2, note 2) p. 148.
6. Mackarness, *op. cit.* (see chap. 1, note 2).
7. Vaughan, W. T., 'Specific Treatment of Hay Fever during the Attack', in *Journal of the American Medical Association*, 80 (Chicago, Illinois, 1925) p. 245.
8. Hansel, F. K., 'Coseasonal Intracutaneous Therapy of Hayfever', in *Journal of Allergy*, 12 (St Louis, Missouri 1941) p. 475.
9. Rinkel, H. J., 'The Management of Clinical Allergy', in *Archives of Otolaryngology*, 76 (Chicago, Illinois, 1962) p. 489.
10. Miller, J. B., *Food Allergy: Provocative Testing and Injection Therapy* (Charles C. Thomas, Springfield, Illinois, 1972).
11. Dickey, L. D., 'Sublingual Use of Allergenic Extracts', in *Otolaryngologic Allergy* (monograph) ed. H. C. King (Elsevier, New York, 1981).

Chapter 6

1. Downing, Dr D., 'For Allergies It's the best Testing System We Have', in *Journal of Alternative Medicine* (West Byfleet, Oct. 1983) pp. 8–10.
2. Tevion, R. J., 'Immunologic Mechanisms in the Production of Food Sensitivities', in *Laryngoscope*, 91 (St Louis, Missouri, 1981) pp. 1913–36.
3. Randolph T. G., 'Hospital Comprehensive Environment Control Program', in Dickey (ed.), *op. cit.* (see chap 2, note 3) pp. 70–85.
4. Ibid.
5. Ibid.
6. Coca, *op. cit.* (see chap. 1, note 1) 1942 edition, p. 15.
7. Ibid.

Chapter 8

1. Newbold, H. L., *Meganutrients for Your Nerves* (Berkley, New York, 1975).
2. Fife, W. S., Professional Drive, Sacramento, CA 95825, *Auto-immune Urine Therapy, An Immunologic Breakthrough for Allergy Related Diseases* (monograph).
3. Dunne, A. P., 'The Use of Injected and Sublingual Urine in the Treatment of Allergies – a Preliminary Report' (essay) (Action Against Allergy, London, 1980).
4. Ibid.
5. Schmidt, H., *Behring-Werke Mitteilungen*, 29 (Marburg, W. Germany, 1954) p. 47.
6. Lerner *et al.*, 'The Introduction of Acute Glomerulonephritis in Rabbits with Soluble Antigens Isolated from Normal Homologous and Autologous Urine', in *Journal of Immunology*, 100 (Baltimore, Maryland, 1968) p. 1277.
8. Purcell, H. M. Jr., 322 West McDowell Rd, Phoenix, Arizona, 'A Hyposensitization Procedure for Nephrosis using an Assumed Antigen Derived from Patient Urine (paper) (American College of Allergists, April 1966).

Chapter 9

1. Lazar, P., 'Hair Analysis; What does it tell us?' in *Journal of the American Medical Association*, 229 (Chicago, Illinois, 1974) p. 1908.
2. Mackenzie, J., 'Alteration of Zinc and Copper Concentration in Hair', in *American Journal of Clinical Nutrition* (Bethesda, Maryland, 1978) pp. 470–6.
3. Kennington, G. S., 'Soluble and Fixed Elements in Mammalian Hair', in *Science*, 155 (Washington, DC, 1967) pp. 588–90.
4. Passwater R. A. and Cranton, E. M., *Trace Elements, Air Analysis and Nutrition* (Keats, New Canaan, Conecticut, 1983).
5. Bryce-Smith, D. and Waldon, H. A., 'Lead, Behaviour and Criminality', in *Ecologist*, 4, No 10 (Camelford, 1974).
6. Schauss, A., *Diet, Disease and Delinquency* (Cancer Control Society, Los Angeles, California).

Chapter 10

1. Mumby, K., *The Food Allergy Plan* (Unwin Paperbacks, London, 1985).
2. Mackarness, *op. cit.* (see chap. 1, note 2).
3. Mandell, *op. cit.* (see chap. 3, note 1) p. 87.
4. Monro, Dr J., *What Agribusiness Does to You*.

Index